MW00769993

STRESS PANDEMIC
9 Natural Steps
To Break The Cycle of Stress & Thrive

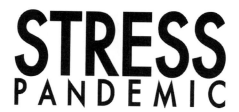

STRESS
PANDEMIC

9 Natural Steps
To Break The Cycle of Stress & Thrive

A Unique LifeReStyle Solution

PAUL HULJICH

Foreword by Hugh Polk, M.D.

www.paulhuljich.com
www.StressPandemic.com
www.LifeReStyle.org
www.mwella.org

Library of Congress Cataloguing-in-Publication Data
PCN: TXu 1-901-209

ISBN 978-0-9848204-0-5

Book design : Jasmine Germani
Typeset in 11/20 Minion

Distributed by Ingram and Midpoint Trade Books, New York
www.midpointtrade.com

Printed in the United States of America

DEDICATION

Stress affects us all in different ways and can lead to serious mind conditions. This book is dedicated to all people who suffer from, or know others who have suffered from, any of the following:

Anxiety

Attention-deficit hyperactivity disorder (ADHD)

Bipolar disorder/manic depression

Compulsive behavior, including addictions to alcohol, recreational or prescription drugs, sex, smoking, gambling, or any other behavior

Depression

Eating disorders, including anorexia and bulimia

Panic attacks

Phobias

Postpartum depression

Post-traumatic stress disorder (PTSD)

Schizophrenia

Seasonal affective disorder (SAD)

Suicide (actual or attempted)

Any other mind condition

CONTENTS

Are you asleep at the wheel?

Are you heading to the edge?

Are you riding a tsunami

and heading for a wipeout?

What are you doing about it?_PH

FOREWORD

Paul Huljich has written a most valuable and helpful book. I agree with him that there is a pandemic of stress: day in and day out we all find ourselves trying to deal with circumstances and situations that may be difficult, painful, bewildering—and, as he amply documents—countless numbers of people around the world are being badly hurt, physically and emotionally, by the stress of it all. Paul was one of those damaged people.

He tells his personal story with great openness and honesty: in the course of becoming the highly successful CEO of a growing company he drove himself to a complete nervous breakdown. In doing so, he was hospitalized with what was diagnosed as bipolar disorder and was told by eminent psychiatrists in New Zealand and the United States that he would need to take psychotropic medications for the rest of his life in order to keep his biomedical disease under control. But Paul refused to accept this grim prognosis. So he set out to build a different, drug-free road for himself—to create a meaningful life, on his own terms but not by himself.

Remarkably, he has succeeded in that goal of creating a joyous and productive life, closely connected to other people— without ever again taking the prescribed medications, without ever having another psychotic episode, without ever needing hospitalization or therapy.

As a traditionally trained psychiatrist who has spent the past thirty-plus years teaching and practicing an alternative therapeutic approach that rejects diagnosing and labeling people in favor of nurturing their growth and development, I'm inspired by what Paul has accomplished and touched by his generosity in wanting to teach others what he has learned in the course of creating his life.

There's a temptation to regard Paul as a hero, someone possessing extraordinary willpower and courage and determination. But I think that misses the most important point of Paul's story, which is that he's a wonderfully ordinary man who day after day, putting one foot in front of the other, kept making little decisions, self-consciously choosing what and when and how he did everything, from getting up in the morning, to eating, to exercising, to responding to things going wrong and even to relating in new ways to his old habits. We learn from what Paul has written that our lives change not as a result of that one, big, apocalyptic moment when we "see the light" but rather through the day-to-day, moment-to-moment small choices we make to do things differently from how we're supposed to do them or how we've always done them before. And we can keep on growing, indefinitely, by continuing to change those little things.

Paul has written a guidebook, an extended set of very practical stage directions, for the rest of us ordinary people to use in performing/creating our own lives.

Given the chaotic, maddening world we live in, I don't think it's possible to eliminate stress entirely from our lives. The key here is not to try to reduce stress by wishing the world were different from what it is but rather to live life productively and joyously *given* that the world is hard to live in, without getting stressed out (of our minds). We have to accept this world—not passively, but actively—by deciding *how* we respond to whatever pain or difficulties we may encounter along the way. Not easy, but Paul is an excellent guide. Happy reading! And pass the book on to others—we can all use this kind of help.

Hugh Polk, M.D.
May 2012

Hugh Polk, M.D., a board-certified psychiatrist, earned his M.D. at Case Western Reserve University. During his more than thirty years of practice as a psychiatrist, he has been the medical director of inpatient psychiatric units and outpatient therapy clinics in New York City. He currently resides and practices in Manhattan.

*I am deeply grateful to all the
wonderful people—especially my son Simon,
and my friend Jasmine—who have spent
many long hours helping me
make this book a reality.*

You are not alone

You are worth it

Have hope

*Never give up.*_{PH}

LETTER TO THE READER

In 2010 I published the novel *Betrayal of Love and Freedom,* a psychological thriller based in part on my own experiences with chronic, unchecked stress and some of its more extreme consequences. Although the novel incorporated some components of the lessons I learned in my journey to wellness, I have long had a desire to share the full body of wisdom that enabled me to transform and restyle my way of life.

The key to my breakthrough was the recognition that stress was the root cause of my problems. I realized that in order to free myself from the serious neurochemical imbalances I had developed, I had to learn how to free myself from harmful stress. I was determined to find a cure and would not take "no" for an answer. Stress can manifest in many different forms and can have serious physical as well as psychological consequences. In my case, unchecked stress manifested at first in physical symptoms and then more seriously in anxiety, severe depression, and ultimately bipolar disorder. As I was told by my doctors, my downward spiral into physical and mental health problems was the result of prolonged stress, primarily in the realms of work and family. It culminated in a full mental breakdown; the results were devastating. On reflection, I could see that I bought into the myth that if I just worked hard enough and attained everything I wished for, I would finally have happiness and peace of mind. My business ambitions, along with my need to please those close to me and maintain harmony at any cost, drove me over the edge.

What began as mild anxiety progressed to crippling depression, mood swings, and bizarre behavior. On the day of my breakdown, I lost all of my rights as a New Zealand citizen and was placed under the control of the state. In the ensuing months, after regaining my rights, I was to spend time at the world-renowned Mayo Clinic and later admit myself for an extended period to the Menninger Clinic in an effort to understand my condition. Ultimately, I would be diagnosed by eleven psychiatrists with what is now known as type 1 bipolar disorder. Each of these doctors cited stress as the cause of my condition and as central to any attempt to deal with it. I was told by my doctors, in no uncertain terms, that there was no cure for bipolar disorder and that I would need to be on medication for the rest of my life.

Despite this prognosis, within two years I was able to free myself from dependence on medication, turn my life around, and enjoy the best years of well-being I have ever experienced. For more than ten years now, I have been completely free of any psychotropic medication, including sleeping tablets. I have had no need for a psychiatrist or therapist and have experienced no symptoms or relapses whatsoever of bipolar disorder, depression, or any other psychological imbalance. Even the psychological crutches and habits I once leaned on to cope with stress no longer have a hold on me. I was able to achieve all this after having been told by doctors that a serious relapse of bipolar disorder was assured within a maximum of seven years.

While speaking with people about my first book and its core message, the most common question I received was, "How did you do it?" I was being asked how I managed to cure myself of bipolar disorder, a condition widely regarded as incurable. The answer, very simply, is this: I learned to master stress. I was told by doctors that the only way I could hope to live a somewhat normal life was by managing the stress in my life. It soon became clear to me that, if I wanted to be free of my condition and still live a full life with all its ups and downs, I would need to go much further than merely managing stress: I would need to master it.

Knowing that the condition I wanted to overcome was purportedly unbeatable, I realized that my success would require experimentation. Thus, I became the guinea pig for my own extensive research, which commenced during my time in the clinics and continued far beyond. Through my own experimentation, I left no stone unturned and gradually developed powerful practices that were able to be incorporated into a busy, full life.

This research and wisdom would eventually be distilled into the Nine Natural Steps that make up the LifeReStyle Solution, though further resources are available at the back of this book, at www.StressPandemic.com, and at our health blog, www.LifeReStyle.org. Although the steps are intentionally simple and have been designed to be easily implemented, it is the synergy of practicing all nine steps in harmony that holds the secret of their power. Moreover, the steps themselves go further than might be suspected at first glance. For example, the nine steps' prescription for "walking" is not the same as what is typically thought of as walking. Instead, it is a brisk, aerobic exercise that also incorporates important silent time for personal reflection and contemplation. Similarly, the requirements of "juicing" are specific and detailed, and this direction's efficacy depends upon these specifics being adhered to.

Indeed, at one time I considered many elements of my previous way of life, leading up to my breakdown, to be healthy. Only in retrospect could I understand that the care I was taking in my well-being was nowhere near enough, given the amount of stress I was subjecting myself to, nor was it balanced as an overall approach to wellness.

Through trial and error, I developed these nine steps drawing on understandings of the brain's neurochemistry. I learned of the five neurochemicals that are central to our wellness: serotonin, epinephrine (or adrenaline), norepinephrine, dopamine, and endorphins. After listening to various doctors tell me of my chemical imbalance I spent years conducting extensive research. These five neurochemicals have a profound effect on our psychological state and also respond directly to our thoughts, feelings, emotions, and moods. Not surprisingly, these are also the neurochemicals typically targeted by major drug companies when developing psychotropic medications.

It is only upon reflection that I realize my neurochemistry was changing as I failed to recognize the significance of the symptoms of stress that I was experiencing. As a businessman, I realized that being able to withstand the stressors of one's career path requires real fortification of oneself, whether you're working as a CEO or in the mailroom. Despite the success that I found in the business world, I found that I was not happy; my life was not balanced, and my health and wellness suffered greatly.

My understanding of the concept of moderation was also rather inaccurate, something that I have come to see is very common. Even more important, I had little awareness of the "transformative" wisdom contained in the first three steps of this book. Once we bring our lives into balance, however, our bodies are capable of rapid healing, and we are able to once again build our resilience. At this time, it is possible for us to relax our routine to a degree and—no longer at the mercy of our addictive tendencies—occasionally enjoy comforts and indulgences that once were harmful to our well-being.

These steps work on two levels. First, they support the health and strength of both body and mind, allowing you to tolerate stress without it taking a heavy toll on your well-being. The second level is more fundamental, and it involves transforming the ways stress is dealt with, enabling you to free yourself from the negative consequences of stress by promoting self-awareness. Because of the holistic nature of the steps and their impact throughout all facets of life, they ultimately work by transforming your lifestyle from one based on unconscious decisions and burdened by stress to one based on self-awareness. The individual ideas in the book are not groundbreaking in themselves, but taken together as a whole, they are a unique approach to complete wellness that draws upon the most powerful tools available.

The synergy of the steps is the source of their power. Too

often we attempt to address our problems in isolation from one another, when the truth is that all of our symptoms are interrelated and that all are related to our psychological and lifestyle choices. Instead of approaching factors such as sleep, coping mechanisms, and excess weight in isolation, the nine steps address the whole context of one's life, addressing imbalances on every level, rather than just on one level. The Nine Natural Steps are about examining your whole life.

Having cured myself of one of the most severe manifestations of stress and having witnessed the stress levels in our world today reaching pandemic levels, I wanted to make my discoveries available to those who might benefit from them and to prevent others from going anywhere near where I went. The world today has become a bit of a bullying place, with stress lurking around every corner. According to the World Health Organization, lifestyle diseases—conditions resulting from one's way of life—have become the leading cause of death in the world today. As I see it, stress is a leading factor in lifestyle disease, as it is caused by the decisions we make in our lives. Poor lifestyle decisions often result from stress, and they can in themselves be the source of further stress in a perpetual, self-reinforcing cycle. I see mind conditions—such as those I suffered from as a result of stress—as lifestyle diseases resulting in large part from our way of life. Unfortunately, many of us only make real changes in our lives when we are forced to, making it significantly more difficult for us to change direction. It has long been a closely held principle of mine that prevention is the key. Ultimately, it is up to us to take responsibility for our way of life, our stress, and our well-being.

Although this book is intended for the many people who deal

with the more common manifestations of stress, I want to be clear that, for those who experience more severe consequences of stress such as depression or bipolar disorder, I am not advocating the immediate withdrawal from all medication. Indeed, in my recovery from bipolar disorder, my withdrawal from reliance on medication was gradual, and I did so very carefully under the supervision of my psychiatrist at the time while also seeking feedback from family and friends. My point is not that we should turn our backs on the help that the medical profession has to offer; it is that the possibility exists for all of us—whether our stress levels are mild or severe—to be free of the burden of stress, and to live fully.

Stress Pandemic contains the practical and powerful keys to breaking the cycle of stress and thriving that I have developed and refined over years of experience and research. It is a book that can be referred back to frequently throughout your journey; indeed, it offers its greatest value when used this way. My hope is that you will keep it somewhere easily accessible—on the bedside table, perhaps—so that it can serve as a constant companion as you fortify and empower yourself.

By implementing these powerful nine natural steps you can break the cycle of stress, take back control of your life, and find contentment, joy, and optimal health.

Paul Huljich
New York, New York
Spring 2014

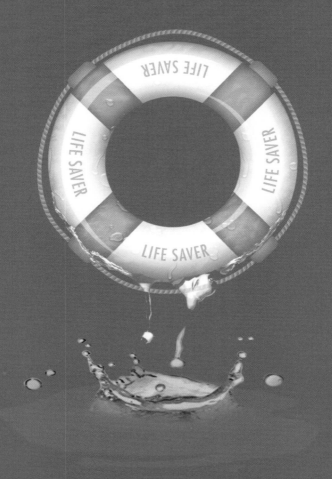

Throw yourself a lifesaver:
break the cycle of stress and thrive.
Paul Huljich

PART ONE

Why Read This Book?

CHAPTER ONE
THE STRESS PANDEMIC

Take control of your stress
before it takes control of you.
Paul Huljich

~~~

Stress is painful. Stress kills. What are you doing about it? Stress has reached pandemic levels and it is affecting everyone; no one is immune to stress and no one escapes its clutches. Yet stress has and always will be a natural part of the human experience. From the day we are born until the day we die, we are faced with challenges and problems. Dealing with these is a part of life; we all experience stress to some degree.

However, the amount of stress we see throughout the world today is abnormal by historical standards and certainly not desirable. In the current information age, stress is seemingly unavoidable. Since the advent of the lightbulb, the way we live has drifted further and further from natural cycles to a point where it is normal for our bodies and minds to be in disharmony.

Global urbanization and the growth of technology have created a world in which access to information has become an obligation and a necessity. People are now held accountable for their actions and whereabouts at all times, and their privacy is jeopardized in ways that were never before possible. We have been invaded by technology on all fronts, and we are often expected to be reachable on our cell phones or by e-mail at all times, even when we attempt to have a vacation. Our personal and work boundaries are blurred to the point where we never experience true downtime anymore.

> *Stress is nothing more than a socially*
> *acceptable form of mental illness.*
> Richard Carlson

Competition in today's world is fierce. What was once enjoyable becomes infused with a sense of fear and urgency, and then it becomes "work" and a task to be dispensed with. Pressure to perform is often intense, and we are constantly evaluated by tests, from early childhood right through our adult working lives. We encounter stress in all domains of our lives: relationships, social interactions, work, career, finances, parenting, health, planning for the future, changes in our environment, war, social upheaval, natural and man-made catastrophes, and our everyday activity.[1] In addition, we are continually under assault on a physical level, with our environment filled with never-before-seen levels of toxicity. From the food we eat to the air we breathe, our bodies are subjected to constant man-made stress as they absorb the toxins that have been introduced to our everyday environment in recent decades, such as artificial food additives, genetically modified organisms (GMOs), Phytoremediation, industrial chemicals, heavy metals, and pharmaceutical residues.

In short, the relentless pace and complexity of modern life has led us to forsake our privacy and our ability to live fully in the present moment. While stress is present in any life to varying degrees, it is now growing into a global problem of serious importance. Even people who wouldn't describe themselves as "being under a lot of stress" still live in this complicated world and still encounter problems and challenges that inevitably give rise to stress.

Stress negatively impacts how we experience our lives by preventing us from living in a state of contentment and fulfillment. Notice for yourself how difficult it is to feel content while you are managing some degree of stress. The truth is, it's not possible. A state of contentment (or happiness, or whatever word we may use to describe a desirable condition) cannot coexist with real stress.

Much of the stress in our lives, however, is not visible. It may be relatively insignificant on a conscious level, and although it limits the fullness to which we can live, we don't notice it or recognize it as a problem. Often, it is only when the grip of stress manifests itself in specific symptoms that stress becomes visible to us. It is at this stage that people may experience substantial physical consequences of prolonged stress. This is also when *mind conditions* may start to arise, beginning with some form of anxiety or depression that can grow into serious mental illness.

Having encountered and naturally cured myself of severe

levels of stress, anxiety, depression, and ultimately bipolar disorder in my own life, I have spent much time studying and researching stress along with what I call *mind conditions*. I use the term *mind conditions* to refer to any serious psychological imbalance, such as depression, anxiety, panic attacks, attention-deficit/hyperactivity disorder (ADHD), post-traumatic stress disorder (PTSD), eating disorders, phobias, or compulsive behavior. In my experience, and from the extensive research I have conducted on the subject, there is a clear and strong link between stress in one's life and the appearance or triggering of mind conditions. Many studies have provided compelling evidence to support what I see as a logical line of cause and effect, i.e., psychological disharmony (stress) leading to potential psychological imbalance (mind conditions).[2] This link has become so clear to me in my observations that I see stress as the basis for almost any mind condition. Consider the following.

According to the World Health Organization (WHO), currently one person in every four develops one or more mental disorders at some stage in life. Today, 450 million people globally suffer from mental disorders in both developed and developing countries.[3] According to the National Institute of Mental Health, an estimated 26.2 percent of Americans age eighteen and older—about one in four adults—suffer from a diagnosable mental disorder in a given year.[4] It is estimated that by 2020, depression will be the second greatest contributor to the global burden of disease.[5] According to the WHO, suicide causes more deaths than homicide or war, with the global suicide rate up 60 percent over the last forty-five years and an even more marked increase in the developed world.[6]

*Stress in life affects everyone and can lead
to serious conditions of the body and mind.*[PH]

Consider the world today and its trends—where we were ten or twenty years ago and where we are now. It isn't hard to see as a general trend that both the everyday and global challenges we face, as well as the demands on our personal time and resources, are only increasing with each passing year. As the statistics on mental health trends demonstrate, the incidence of mental illness is rising sharply—evidence of the growing toll that stress is taking on our lives.

This is what I mean when I refer to the *stress pandemic* that our global society is experiencing today. Moreover, the existence of a stress pandemic in our world will only become more obvious in coming years, given current trends. The question is, do we want our lives to be dominated by stress, and if not, what are we doing about it?

Stress and poor lifestyle choices

can be the root of all evil,

relentlessly looking for a weakness

in the mind and body.

We often deal with the symptoms of stress,

not the causes.

*Master stress and live well.*PH

POTENTIAL EFFECTS OF STRESS
Do you suffer from any of the following?

- Frequent headaches, jaw clenching or pain
- Gritting, grinding teeth
- Stuttering or stammering
- Tremors, trembling of lips/hands
- Neck ache, back pain, muscle spasms
- Light headedness, faintness, dizziness
- Ringing, buzzing, or "popping" sounds
- Frequent blushing, sweating
- Cold or sweaty hands, feet
- Dry mouth, problems swallowing
- Frequent colds, infections, herpes sores
- Rashes, itching, hives, "goose bumps"
- Unexplained or frequent "allergy" attacks
- Heartburn, stomach pain, nausea
- Excess belching, flatulence
- Constipation, diarrhea
- Difficulty breathing, sighing
- Sudden attacks of panic
- Chest pain, palpitations
- Frequent urination
- Poor sexual desire or performance
- Excess anxiety, worry, guilt, nervousness
- Increased anger, frustration, hostility
- Depression, frequent or wild mood swings
- Increased or decreased appetite
- Insomnia, nightmares, disturbing dreams
- Difficulty concentrating, racing thoughts
- Trouble learning new information
- Forgetfulness, disorganization, confusion
- Difficulty in making decisions
- Feeling overloaded or overwhelmed
- Frequent crying spells or suicidal thoughts
- Feelings of loneliness or worthlessness
- Little interest in appearance, punctuality
- Nervous habits, fidgeting, feet tapping
- Increased frustration, irritability, edginess
- Overreaction to petty annoyances
- Increased number of minor accidents
- Obsessive or compulsive behavior
- Reduced work efficiency or productivity
- Lies or excuses to cover up poor work
- Rapid or mumbled speech
- Excessive defensiveness or suspiciousness
- Problems in communication, sharing
- Social withdrawal and isolation
- Constant tiredness, weakness, fatigue
- Frequent use of over-the-counter drugs
- Weight gain or loss without diet
- Increased smoking, alcohol or drug use
- Excessive gambling or impulse buying

Source : American Stress Institute: www.stress.org

As demonstrated above, stress can have wide-ranging effects on emotions, mood, and behavior. If this list applies to you, please keep reading.

It is not stress alone that kills us;

it is our reaction to it. [PH]

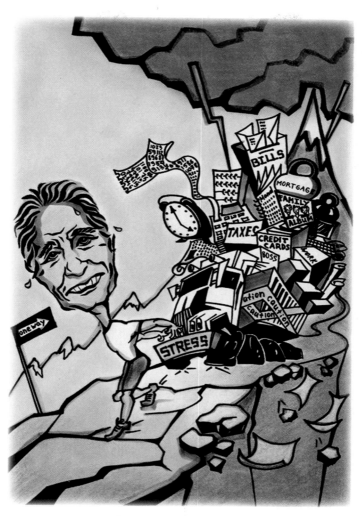

Stress can run you over.

Stress Response : Is the trigger action, when we feel

threatened or challenged and causes a psychological

and physiological change known as the Fight or Flight

reaction; if activated too often will cause serious

*conditions of the mind and the body.*PH

~nae~

CHAPTER TWO

STRESS AND YOU

Sometimes when people are under stress,
they hate to think, and it's the time
when they most need to think.
Bill Clinton

Life is full of frustrations, deadlines, demands, overstimulation, and pressure. As previously mentioned, stress is inevitable in some form or another. Our modern way of life is a breeding ground for stress, and very few, if any, of us are immune.

The human body has evolved to react to stress in ways meant to protect us from predators and other aggressors that posed very real immediate threats throughout our evolutionary history. Such threats are rare today, but that doesn't mean that life is free of stress. On the contrary, most people face multiple demands each day, such as shouldering a huge workload, making ends meet, and taking care of family members. The body often treats such challenges as threats, and as a result you may feel as if you're constantly under assault. But you have a choice; you don't have to let stress control your life.

The Stress Response

The stress response is the psychological and physiological reaction that is triggered when you feel threatened or challenged, giving rise to the fight-or-flight mode. In many of us the stress response is active much of the time, throwing our bodies and minds off balance.

The body's stress response is natural, a physiological reaction that is triggered in the presence of perceived threats. When one senses danger—real or imagined—the body's defense system kicks into a rapid, automatic process known as the fight-or-flight reaction, or the stress response. The nervous system responds by stimulating the release of a flood of neurochemicals and hormones, primarily epinephrine, norepinephrine, and cortisol. These neurochemicals and hormones rouse the body for emergency action. Senses become sharper, the heart rate increases, muscles tighten, blood pressure rises, the air passage constricts and breath quickens. There is a metabolic shift on a cellular level. This state of alert is designed to decrease reaction time and enhance focus, speed, and stamina—all in preparation for either fighting off or fleeing from the danger at hand.

The stress response is helpful in emergency situations, in certain immediate challenges that we face in life, and for situations where heightened performance is required. However, what is unnatural and dangerous is stress that is not generated for any immediate situation but instead underlies our everyday life because we have failed to examine and deal with it. This kind of unnatural stress serves no purpose but to damage our health, our productivity, our relationships, and our experience of life. The human body does not differentiate between our overreaction to life's ups and downs versus a life-or-death situation; it responds in the same way to both. Therefore, if you are frequently worried and feeling under pressure, your emergency stress response may be switched on much of the time. The body exhibits warning signs when you are suffering from an unhealthy amount of stress, which can manifest not only on a physical level but also emotionally, behaviorally, and cognitively. Much like a car's glowing "check engine" light, neglecting these warning signs can cause a major malfunction.

Good Stress versus Bad Stress

So called "good stress," sometimes referred to as "eustress," is the type of stress we feel when excited. This stress response to some kind of "play" accelerates our pulse and alters our neurochemical and hormonal balance, but we don't perceive any real threat or fear. We may feel this type of temporary stress while enjoying a game of tennis, riding a roller coaster, or going on a first date. This good stress arises in many scenarios and it keeps us feeling alive and excited about life.

There are two main forms of "bad stress": acute stress and chronic stress. Acute stress is triggered by trauma or terror, activating an immediate and severe stress response. Such events may include life-or-death situations, witnessing horrific events, or experiencing trauma such as rape or attack, to name a few.

The type of stress that we are typically most challenged by, and with which this book is concerned, is chronic stress. When we repeatedly face stressors that take a heavy toll on us over time and that feel inescapable chronic stress results. Like a tap that's left running and is never turned off, we deplete our energy and resources. The ways in which we create this form of stress are many, from the circumstantial triggers such as work life, home life, and logistics, to those that rest more upon our emotional and thought patterns. Acute stress can also easily give rise to chronic stress once the initial traumatic event has passed.

Sources of Stress

Some people experience mild or moderate stress continuously and become accustomed to it, never actually noticing its impact or having their responses to stress put to the test by prolonged and intense challenges. There are others who are simply more adept at handling stress and not letting it control them, by virtue of their natural disposition and personality traits. For most of us, however, stress plays an important role in our lives—even if we have yet to truly appreciate its impact—and its effects on us are both psychological and physical.

Whether it's the logistical pressure we feel in trying to organize our busy lives and fulfill duties and obligations each day or whether it's stress in the emotional realm of fear, worry, anxiety, regret, guilt, confusion, and anger, stress takes its toll on our mind and body. In today's world, most of us, to some degree, deal with a sense of feeling overwhelmed by daily responsibilities and challenges, knowing that we can't possibly accomplish everything that we think we need to get done. Even when certain tasks are pleasurable or exciting, a sense of anxiety still exists over our commitments that may involve hard choices, disappointing others, or letting go of an objective we are anxious to complete. It may also be that procrastination and resistance to doing the work we know needs to be done creates its own kind of anxiety, even when there's no sense of rushing to complete it all. Similarly, the emotional stresses of life—in varying degrees—are unavoidable and are part of the experience of growing up and passing through different stages of life, having relationships of different kinds, and encountering changes, challenges, and loss.

While chronic stress is most often caused by ongoing psychological tension in response to the pressures of life, it is also possible for continuous physiological and environmental stressors to result in chronic stress. For example, a person suffering from a chronic illness can develop chronic stress in response to the physical pain, discomfort, and depleted energy levels related to her illness. Similarly, the challenges to our physical well-being to which we are exposed on a daily basis as a result of our modern lifestyles—such as pollutants of all kinds and poor dietary, sleep, and exercise patterns—stress our bodies and our ability to deal with life and experience wellness. This, in turn, can increase our stress levels and contribute to chronic stress.

Stress is relative, and we all experience stress in different ways, with each of us having our own level of tolerance for stress. Similarly, we each react differently to different sources of stress. Sources of stress vary and include everything from family issues and bereavement to issues of financial security and career.

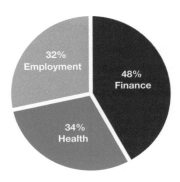

A 2006 study by Mental Health America found that 48% of American adults were stressed by finances, 34% by health issues, and 32% by employment issues, with parents reporting the greatest amount of stress out of any demographic group.[7] Stress can arise from the pressures created by having too much to do in the limited time we have each day while we struggle to create time for our own enjoyment, rest, and self-care.

So much stress is avoided
*when we manage our time more wisely.*_{PH}

Stress is intricately linked to our emotional life and thought patterns, with the disharmony of anger, fear, and the whole spectrum of emotional experience generating a near constant stream of stress for some people. Even something as seemingly harmless as noisy neighbors can be a significant source of stress in a person's life.

Stress in the Workplace

Occupational stress has been defined as a "global epidemic" by the United Nations' International Labor Organization, one that has alarming physical, psychological, and economic consequences. With three out of four Americans describing their work as stressful, and almost one in three reporting high levels of stress at work, occupational stress costs U.S. employers an estimated $300 billion per year in lower productivity, absenteeism, staff turnover, workers' compensation, medical insurance and other stress-related expenses.[8]

Job-related stress comes in different forms and affects wellness in various ways. We're all aware of the small things that can irritate us, such as the crashing computer or ceaselessly ringing phones, while major stress can arise from having too much or not enough work to do or from doing work in which you find very little meaning. Conflicts with clients, coworkers, or superiors are, of course, other major sources of stress, as are taking on extra responsibilities and feeling undercompensated for the work that you do. Feeling as if you have no control over your work or job duties is the biggest cause of occupational stress, and people who feel that they have no control at work are most likely to get stress-related illnesses. If you don't find enough meaning in your job, this can impair your overall performance and in turn lead to your feeling insecure about your job performance, another major source of stress for many people in the work place. Lastly, poor communication, lack of support from your boss or colleagues, and dangerous or unpleasant working conditions add fuel to the bonfire of unrelenting stress that can be found on the job.

Major corporations have recognized that stress management training can be very cost effective. It reduces employee absenteeism, work injuries, health costs, and worker turnover.

It also improves quality, productivity, and harmony. Consider the following U.S. examples of the impact of stress on business:

- A million workers per day are estimated to miss work due to stress problems.
- 60 to 80% of all industrial accidents are due to stress.
- 40% of employee turnover is due to job stress.
- Workplace violence is skyrocketing with about a million non-fatal violent crimes occurring each year in the workplace. Murder is now the second highest cause of occupational fatalities among both sexes, and the leading cause for females, with an average of twenty workers murdered each week.[9]

Stress causes poor lifestyle choices
Poor lifestyle choices cause stress
*It is a self-perpetuating cycle*_{PH}

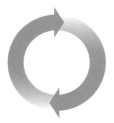

Awareness of Stress During Pregnancy

Even the physiology of children and fetuses in the womb can be affected by stress. For example, if a fetus is traumatized by its carrier, its cortisol level is likely to increase and impair the neuronal growth of the baby, and babies exposed to postpartum depression (also known as postnatal depression) are more likely to have elevated cortisol levels during adolescence, affecting their temperament.[10]

While a child is still in its mother's womb, the brain's neuronal system is wired into billions of connections like a vast tapestry—as many stars as there are in the Milky Way. During this vulnerable time, the mother's physical and emotional well-being can have profound effects upon the development of the fetus. As with alcohol, smoking and drug use affect the fetus and elevated cortisol levels in the mother have been found to have significant consequences for newborns.[11] Research has shown that from birth to the age of eight months, babies are growing increasingly aware of the sounds, tastes, smells, and sights around them. During this process, the number of neurons in the brain continues to increase up until the age of three.[12,13] A child that grows up in a happy environment exhibits normal cortisol levels, but if the child is traumatized by its carrier, the cortisol levels are elevated which impairs the child's neuronal growth after birth. Furthermore, a child born with elevated levels of cortisol is typically less tolerant and more easily upset and distracted.[14] Thus, parents of an unborn child should have a greater awareness of their lifestyle, as it can negatively impact the unborn child's development.

Colostrum is the "first milk", also known colloquially as beestings or bisnings. It is a form of milk produced by the mammary glands of humans (mammals). It gives the newborn child immunity to infection by providing the antibodies it needs. It also helps in passing the first bowel motion, by stimulating the gastrointestinal or GI tract. Bacteria present in breast milk constitutes one of the initial instances of contact with microorganisms that colonies the infant's digestive system, introducing the first probiotic bacteria to our gut system. Research shows that breast milk bacteria is important for the development of the immune system. The lack of colostrum could increase the possibilities of allergies, asthma and autoimmune diseases. Colostrum, could be beneficial for the treatment of a wide variety of gastrointestinal conditions, drug-induced gut injury, and chemotherapy-induced mucosites.[15]

It is very important to have an awareness of the necessity to help fortify your newborn child, by providing the infant with the 'tools to survive' the stress pandemic and thrive.

Stress and You

Prolonged and constant stress can lead to serious health problems, as chronic unchecked stress disrupts nearly every system in the body. It can raise blood pressure, suppress the immune system (or, alternatively, lead to autoimmune diseases), cause inflammation, worsen allergies,[16] increase the risk of heart attack and stroke, impair fertility, and accelerate the aging process.[17] Stress, and the unhealthy lifestyle choices that often follow from stress and a lack of awareness, can also be looked upon as a major factor in "lifestyle diseases." For example, the Mental Health America study found that 37% of adult Americans turn to eating as a coping mechanism for stress, while 26% turn to smoking, drinking, or drugs.[18] The WHO reports that lifestyle diseases now account for 63 percent of global deaths based on its estimates for 2008.[19]

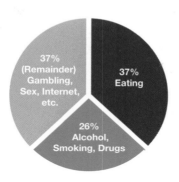

Beyond these physical stress-related complications, stress is the basic foundation of many psychological imbalances. These may also be viewed as lifestyle diseases, their root cause being traceable to the experience of stress—which can sensibly be regarded as a lifestyle factor. Early symptoms of moderate to high levels of stress include: sleeping difficulties; worry; teeth-grinding; limited patience; high irritability; abiding feelings of sadness, anxiety, or depression; absence of contentment or joy; lack of energy; and difficulties with concentration.

Stress is to the human being as rust is to the car: corrosive and destructive.₍PH₎

Eventually, mind conditions can develop. These conditions are observable from a physiological standpoint in the imbalance of the brain's neurochemistry. The six most important neurochemicals linked to personality, thoughts, feelings, emotions, and moods are serotonin, epinephrine, dopamine, endorphins, norepinephrine, and melatonin.

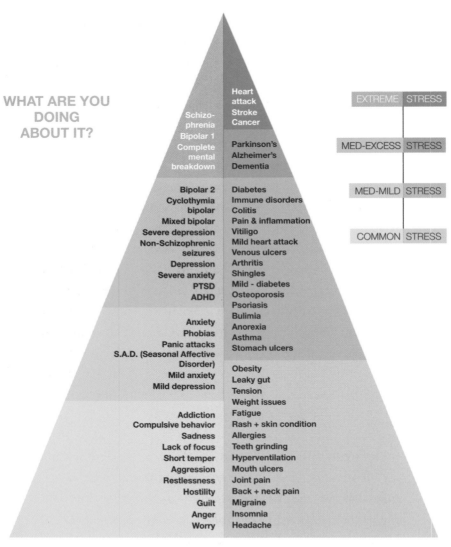

LifeReStyle Solution
Pyramid of Stress
Symptoms & Consequences of Stress
Warning Signs

WHAT ARE YOU
DOING
ABOUT IT?

EXTREME STRESS

MED-EXCESS STRESS

MED-MILD STRESS

COMMON STRESS

Schizo-
phrenia
Bipolar 1
Complete
mental
breakdown

Heart
attack
Stroke
Cancer

Parkinson's
Alzheimer's
Dementia

Bipolar 2
Cyclothymia
bipolar
Mixed bipolar
Severe depression
Non-Schizophrenic
seizures
Depression
Severe anxiety
PTSD
ADHD

Diabetes
Immune disorders
Colitis
Pain & inflammation
Vitiligo
Mild heart attack
Venous ulcers
Arthritis
Shingles
Mild - diabetes
Osteoporosis
Psoriasis

Anxiety
Phobias
Panic attacks
S.A.D. (Seasonal Affective
Disorder)
Mild anxiety
Mild depression

Bulimia
Anorexia
Asthma
Stomach ulcers

Obesity
Leaky gut
Tension
Weight issues

Addiction
Compulsive behavior
Sadness
Lack of focus
Short temper
Aggression
Restlessness
Hostility
Guilt
Anger
Worry

Fatigue
Rash + skin condition
Allergies
Teeth grinding
Hyperventilation
Mouth ulcers
Joint pain
Back + neck pain
Migraine
Insomnia
Headache

Psychological
(Mental / Emotional)

Physiological
(Physical)

Stress Causes Pain in the Mind & Body

"Prevention is far better than recovery"

Stress disrupts neural circuits and can eventually cause serious imbalances in these neurochemicals. These imbalances are closely associated with the presence of mind conditions.[20] Indeed, it is usually these neurochemicals that drug companies target in attempting to treat mind conditions, such as depression, although such approaches to treating mental imbalance typically only address the symptoms rather than the cause of the problem.

Prevention is the key
Prevention is better than recovery.[PH]

We can witness the effects of stress on our psychological well-being by examining the impact of the stress response on some of our most important neurotransmitters. For example, serotonin, which serves to elevate our mood, can become depleted with chronic stress and anxiety. This leaves a person feeling depressed. It also affects the natural sleep cycle by impacting production of melatonin, a hormone central to our circadian rhythms. The balance of dopamine—which is crucial to our experience of pleasure, desire, enjoyment, and motivation—can also be disrupted by excessive stress. Eventually, serious mind conditions, such as depression, anxiety, bipolar disorder, schizophrenia, phobias, panic attacks, post-traumatic stress disorder, eating disorders, ADHD, and compulsive behavior may develop.[21]

Additionally, our neurochemistry can become increasingly imbalanced and potentially toxic as a result of factors related to our chosen lifestyle, such as poor diet and insufficient sleep or exercise.

Stress in moderation isn't always bad; it may be helpful in motivating us to perform under pressure. Yet, when we are operating in emergency mode for a prolonged period, our mind and body pay the price. Moreover, what is often overlooked is the possibility of living a life free of the negative effects of stress. It *is* possible to live a life of fulfillment and contentment, despite the increasingly stressful world we live in.

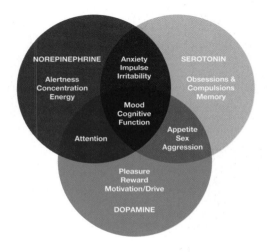

All my life I have tried to
pluck a thistle and plant a flower,
wherever the flower would grow in
thought and mind.
Abraham Lincoln[22]

(Abraham Lincoln, arguably America's greatest and most
loved president, sadly suffered from bipolar disorder)

You gain strength, and courage, and confidence

by every experience in which

you really stop to look fear in the face...

you must do the thing you think you cannot do.

Eleanor Roosevelt

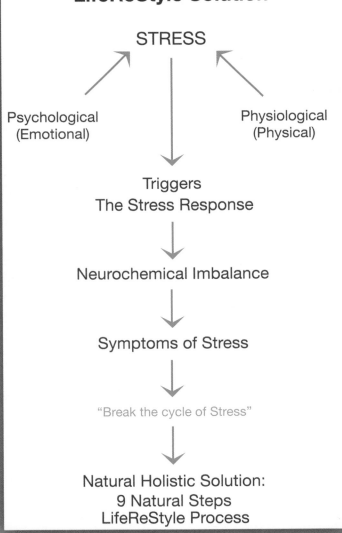

POTENTIAL CAUSES OF STRESS
(in no particular order)

- Death of a loved one
- Divorce or relationship separation
- Injury, illness, or ailment (of the body or mind), or that of a loved one
- Marriage
- Pregnancy
- Gaining of new family member, including through adoption
- Sex
- Dating
- Job change (loss or gain)
- Workplace stress, including: change in/difficult work hours or conditions; trouble with boss; change in job responsibilities
- Making a major financial commitment
- Financial issues, including: debt obligations; loan/mortgage foreclosure; loss of home; bankruptcy; change in financial position/status; tax burden/issues
- Arguments with loved one(s)
- Abuse – physical, verbal, or emotional
- Family member leaving home
- Trouble with family (including in-laws)
- Forced revision of personal habits
- Dealing with addictions or obsessions
- Moving home
- Undesired living situation
- Traffic
- Anticipation of change; for example, first day of new job/school, etc.
- Poor sleep
- Time pressures
- Poor diet
- Not meeting goals, ambitions, or expectations
- Holidays/vacations, including Christmas, Thanksgiving, etc.
- Social affairs/responsibilities
- Legal problems or violations of the law, and potential problems including: resulting financial burden; incarceration
- Retirement
- Onset or sudden gaining of disability
- Stress from sources that may not be assumed to affect many of us but, as time and experience shows, can reach further than we might often think: environmental disasters, (including tsunamis, hurricanes, floods, earthquakes, fires, droughts); civil unrest, war, and/or displacement and after-effects of such; famine; being a victim of crime (for example burglary, assault, blackmail/extortion)
- Stress from sources that may perhaps seem less significant but can take an unexpected toll: noisy neighbors, including infants or pets; loss of personal belongings, particularly valuables; lack of access to nature

(Source: Built upon the references contained in the Surgeon General Mental Health Report on Health: Chapter 4. www.surgeongeneral.gov/library/mentalhealth /chapter4/sec1_1.htm)

The above are potential causes of stress, some major and others seemingly less so. As can be seen, the potential causes of stress are limitless. The key however, is being able to identify them and deal with them accordingly.

Adopting the right attitude

can convert a

negative stress into a positive one.

Hans Hugo Bruno Selye

CHAPTER THREE

BREAKING THE CYCLE OF STRESS

Amidst the rush of worldly comings and goings,
observe how endings become beginnings.
Lao-tzu

W hy is it that most of us are unable to break the cycle of stress? Given that stress is reaching pandemic levels in our world, and considering that stress harms our mind and body and inhibits our ability to live fully, the natural question to ask is, what are you doing about it?

Our first response may be to do our best to avoid stress altogether. Alas, on closer examination, this strategy is not as easy as it seems. It is very difficult to simply say, "I'm not going to have stress in my life." For one thing, even the most luxurious or seemingly carefree environments are still quite capable of causing stress; the human mind will find something to worry about regardless of the situation, as water finds its way into a crevasse. More important, withdrawing from the ups and downs of life is no answer to the problem of stress. It's true that you may limit your exposure to stressors, but in doing so you will also be limiting your experience of the fullness of life. We are supposed to experience both the good and the bad, to learn, to make decisions, to do what we enjoy. There is no reason to give up on the challenge of life when you understand that it is possible to live in balance.

To this point, a serious concern of mine is the growing dependence on psychotropic drugs for the long-term (and often indefinite) treatment of mind conditions. To illustrate, the amount spent on psychotropic drugs in the United States grew from an estimated $2.8 billion in 1987 to nearly $18 billion in 2001, and by as early as 1996 psychotropic drugs were used in 77 percent of mental health treatment cases. Perhaps more worrisome is that, between 1991 and 2006, the use of psychotropic drugs by girls and boys under the age of twenty increased by 300 percent.[23]

*Don't apply a Band-Aid to your challenges and problems; face them head on.*PH

While a pill might potentially alleviate sufferers of mind conditions in the short run, it is not a true solution to the underlying cause of the condition, which is stress of some sort that has not been dealt with. A dependence on avoiding stress in this way is a mask, not a cure, and will only serve to perpetuate the mind condition, leaving the individual wondering if she is truly being herself or if who she is now is partly the result of a drug. Once a period of change is implemented with real commitment to a new way of life, a person can build the strength needed to confront whatever may have led to the development of a mind condition. He or she can then learn to live in balance without dependence on drugs. This way of life is exceedingly more enjoyable, and it soon becomes clear that if we are patient and dedicated, there is no reason to live in fear and avoidance of life's challenges.

*Pause for a moment and reflect on where you are in your life right now and where you are heading.*_{PH}

Preparation and Response

I have discovered that we can beat stress by being committed to real change in two areas of our lives. First, we must prepare ourselves both mentally and physically to be able to withstand stress without it overwhelming us. This aspect of our commitment to wellness involves building and maintaining a daily routine that nourishes and cleanses both mind and body, ensuring that we are better equipped to meet the inevitable challenges of life. The second component concerns our *response to stress.* It is important to note the contrast between this term, *response to stress,* and the fight-or-flight state, called the *stress response.* Whereas our habitual and immediate reaction to a threat or challenge may be the *stress response* (fight-or-flight reaction), the key to well-being lies in our ability to *respond to stress.* We have a choice in how we react to challenges and to stress. When I speak of freeing ourselves from stress, I am referring to both our preparation for dealing with challenges and our chosen responses to them.

These two components—preparation and response—are the essence of the Nine Natural Steps to breaking the cycle of stress and achieving complete wellness.

Take charge; fortify and empower yourself.

You will feel in control

as your ambitions, goals, and desires

*merge with contentment.*_{PH}

CHAPTER FOUR

THE LIFEReSTYLE PROCESS
Nine Natural Steps to
Break the Cycle of Stress

Unchecked stress has very real consequences![PH]

~~~

Before delving into the nine steps of the LifeReStyle Process and their application, I would like to provide a brief background on my experience with stress and how I came to develop the Nine Natural Steps. A fuller account of my experience with stress, addictions, anxiety, depression, and bipolar disorder and my subsequent success in overcoming stress and my stress-related mind conditions using the Nine Natural Steps can be found in Part Three of this book.

> *Opportunities to find deeper powers within oneself*
> *come when life seems most challenging.*
> Joseph Campbell

I have had extensive, firsthand experience with both stress and its dire consequences, as well as with approaches to overcome stress and recover from its effects. It is this experience, as well as the vast research and investigation I conducted during my own painful battle with stress-related imbalance, that gave rise to the development of the Nine Natural Steps for mastering stress. Although I am not a medical doctor or a psychotherapist, I believe that my experience, combined with extensive study, has provided me with rare insight into stress and the recovery from its most dreadful effects.

After many years working toward my ambitions of abundance for myself and for those I loved, I eventually found myself in a position of having everything I had dreamed of. As chairman and joint-CEO of Best Corporation, a company that I had founded with my two brothers, I had pioneered high-quality and organic foods in New Zealand and Australia beginning in the 1980s. We had built Best into a highly successful publicly traded company that we eventually sold to a multinational food corporation. I had achieved what some might think of as the ideal, successful life. I was living in a newly built home that I had designed for my wife, my three sons, and myself—it was the house of my dreams and happened to be the largest ever built in New Zealand at the time. I owned sports cars, a luxury yacht, and we regularly enjoyed lavish vacations. I had realized my dream of building a successful food company and producing something that I believed in, all while being my own boss.

However, it was at this time of apparent success that I began to become aware that there was something wrong with me. It wasn't a physical ailment but a psychological one that had its roots in the severe levels of stress I was experiencing.

Regardless of any level of success I achieved, any resulting sense of satisfaction or joy proved fleeting and left me feeling despondent and wanting more. Although I experienced moments of peace of mind, happiness, and contentment, they were very short-lived and often overcome by anxiety and a dull, flat feeling in my chest and stomach. What was happening unbeknownst to me was occurring physiologically inside myself.

My brain's neurochemistry was becoming more and more disrupted every day, due to the burden of stress in my life. In an effort to address the imbalance in my neurochemistry, I had been seeing a psychiatrist for a number of months who had prescribed antidepressants. However, the effects of the amount of stress I had subjected myself to ultimately proved too great. Like a volcano that blew its top, I eventually suffered a full mental breakdown. I was declared of "unsound mind," made a ward of the state, and diagnosed with bipolar disorder. I was told by multiple doctors—in New Zealand, at the world-renowned Mayo Clinic in Minnesota, and at the Menninger Clinic in Kansas—that there was no cure for bipolar disorder and that I would be dependent on medication for the rest of my life.

However, I was not satisfied with the answers I was given. I could not accept that there was no cure for my condition. I was determined to find some way to rediscover my true self; I was determined to break free from my "chemical straitjacket," as I often referred to the reliance on psychotropic medication. I searched relentlessly for a cure and for answers as to why I was suffering from this condition. I researched mind conditions, I spoke to every doctor I could, and I interviewed fellow patients at the Menninger Clinic in Topeka, Kansas, where I spent six weeks trying to understand and move through my condition.

I was told by various doctors that the only way I could live a somewhat normal life was to carefully manage my stress. To add to the challenge, I was facing not only the accumulated stress of the years that led me to my breakdown in the first place but also the new stress and pressure of living with the stigma and uncertainty of a mind condition. The task before me was to master stress, as well as to strengthen my body and mind to a point where I would be free of my condition.

The Origins of the Nine Natural Steps

Through trial and error, through research into all facets of health, and through interviewing and speaking with whomever I could find to talk to about health, I began to develop processes to rebuild myself. These processes would eventually be refined and organized into the Nine Natural Steps.

The first challenge was to understand the true cause of my illness. There were a variety of factors I could point to, such as the emotional stress and pain I had experienced for many years due to serious ongoing family issues that remain unresolved even today, as well as the pressure and demands of running a thriving business. However, the one understanding that made all the difference was to recognize that it was the "old me," the "old Paul," that got me into this mess. This meant accepting that if I wanted to live fully again and beat my condition, I had to change myself. I had to be proactive in stripping myself back to the core of who I was and then rebuilding myself from scratch. I had to create a new Paul—one who wouldn't make himself sick, a person who would be able to experience life in its full wonder.

I realized that many parts of the person I had become were formed by habit. In this respect, it became very clear to me that my illness was in fact a "lifestyle disease"; it was a direct result of my accumulated conscious and unconscious decisions about the way I lived my life. When my stress response was triggered, I reacted by making poor lifestyle decisions which in turn created greater stress in a perpetual cycle that was harmful to my neurochemical balance. I came to understand that many habits are formed over a thirty-day period of repetition and that these habits shape our lives. Therefore, to deprogram my body and mind of harmful habits, I had to be disciplined about aiming for thirty consecutive days of overriding old habits by learning new ones. Like a child learning to walk, I had to start from the beginning.

It took almost two years for me to develop and implement the Nine Natural Steps and to use this lifestyle approach to overcome my stress and mind conditions, freeing myself from the need for psychotropic medication to balance my neurochemistry. Every doctor I had spoken with had told me that I would suffer from bipolar disorder and be dependent on medication for my entire life. Despite this "life sentence," I succeeded in beating my conditions. Furthermore, it was my goal not only to free myself of medication but also to free myself from the pain and agony of bipolar disorder and depression, as well as the stress that caused them. I didn't want to just treat the symptoms of my problems; I wanted to address the root cause and cure myself completely of these conditions. The Nine Natural Steps enabled me to achieve this.

These nine steps are my approach for managing stress in one's life. It is an approach that has been proven under the toughest circumstances: This is the method that I used to recover from bipolar disorder, a condition widely and firmly believed to be unbeatable. The Nine Natural Steps enabled me to cure myself of all components of my depression and bipolar disorder and to master the underlying cause of these imbalances—stress. It was my success in beating stress that allowed me to do the "impossible" and free myself from serious mind conditions.

Stress is everywhere, and it is inescapable. This book is for people who realize that they have stress in their life to some degree but who have decided that they don't want to be controlled by it. All of us have a right to live life fully and in a state of contentment. No matter what amount of stress you may be experiencing—whether it's everyday stress or whether you have a stress-related condition—the nine steps of the LifeReStyle Process will empower you to fortify yourself, beat stress, and transform your life.

Using the Nine Natural Steps

Part Two contains the nine steps that, when practiced with commitment, provide a means for freeing yourself from harmful stress and recovering from any of the consequences of stress you may be experiencing in your life. Each step is practical and designed to be applied in daily life. This is the purpose of the summary and the questions at the end of each step: to encourage daily or weekly self-assessment, reminders, and further examination of your application of the steps. The questions at the end of each chapter, when approached honestly, are particularly effective. It is useful to return often to the ending questions of each step, using them as tools for transformation by sitting with them and seeing what your honest answers are. In this way, further opportunities for progress can be revealed.

As mentioned earlier, I recommend keeping this book somewhere readily accessible so that you can continue to refer back to the steps throughout your journey. These steps are not designed to be read only once and then put to one side; they are infused with power by your continual interaction with them. The questions at the end of each step are an excellent tool for continual engagement with the steps.

The LifeReStyle Process could be looked upon as a lifestyle solution to stress and its consequences. A "lifestyle" disease, the increasing prevalence of which has already been mentioned, is any disease—physical or psychological—whose cause can be traced to lifestyle decisions. Stress, in turn, is a lifestyle factor, considering that harmful amounts of it are preventable if a balanced way of life and attitude are adopted. This balance is what the Nine Natural Steps offer: By following the LifeReStyle Process, both the psychological and practical aspects of your life are brought into balance, enabling you to enjoy a life unencumbered by harmful stress. Your improved overall wellness and strength will mean that you are also less susceptible to other illnesses and lifestyle-related conditions. An added benefit is that as you begin to eliminate stress from your life, you will find that many of the habitual poor lifestyle decisions of the past naturally become easier to let go of, as many of these choices are, themselves, a result of stress. Many poor lifestyle decisions—such as poor diet, lack of exercise and sleep, and toxic habits such as smoking—are made in an attempt to unconsciously deal with the experience of stress. **The root cause of the cycle of stress begins with the over-activation of the stress response and the resulting disruption of a healthy neurochemical balance. If this imbalance is prolonged, the symptoms of stress will emerge to alert and challenge you.**

Each step is written with an emphasis on practicality and the application of each step's wisdom, rather than lengthy explanations. This approach makes it easy to read and reread each step as needed, with in-depth scientific explanations and references included at the end of the book. A glossary and appendices can be found at the back of the book, while additional resources are available at www.StressPandemic.com and www.LifeReStyle.org.

Over time, you will gain an awareness that you are letting go and adjusting your present lifestyle, as the new lifestyle habits start to take hold in you. This is what I call ReStyling yourself.

*Let each one of us become a leader, not a follower.*_{PH}

The Transformative Steps

Steps 1, 2, and 3 are the transformative steps, designed to address the underlying habits that are the cause of stress. While these steps are essential, they are also steps that you will master gradually and continuously. They are not activities that you can engage in and then move on with the rest of your

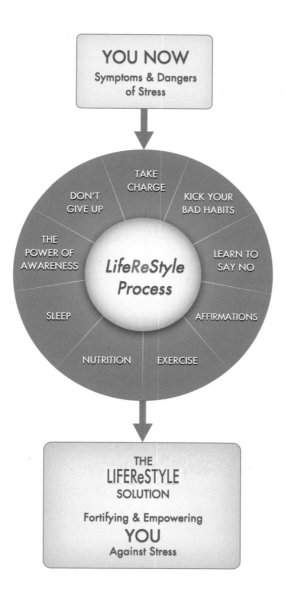

day; they are tools that enable you to shift your attitudes and overcome the causes of stress and, as such, require continual practice, exploration, and development. You will get better and better at using these tools the more you apply them on a day-to-day basis. Eventually, your awareness of these steps becomes tuned so that you are effortlessly and skillfully incorporating these steps into your life as an extension of yourself, as if you are simply breathing. These first three steps are the keys to true personal transformation.

The Practical Steps

Steps 4, 5, 6, and 7 are the practical steps. The function of these steps is to optimize your general wellness and allow you to feel better than you've ever felt before. By strengthening body and mind, they enable you to deal more effectively with stress, assist in the release of stress both physiologically and psychologically, and help maintain a healthy neurochemical balance. These steps also support the development of the first three steps, help to minimize the over-activation of the stress response, and mitigate the symptoms of stress. They can be integrated into your daily routine and then tailored to your particular needs. For example, during periods of greater pressure and stress, you may find yourself needing to be extra vigilant about daily stretching and avoiding all C.R.A.P. (caffeine, refined sugars and sweeteners, alcohol, and processed foods and drinks). However, if you have built the practical steps into your daily routine and after some time find yourself not needing to stretch every day, for instance, it may be appropriate to modify your practice so that you are stretching only two to four times a week during less challenging times. After you have already succeeded in implementing the practical steps into your daily routine, use your judgment in assessing what is best for you.

The Self-Assessment Steps

The final two steps, 8 and 9, provide insight for your continual self-assessment and also serve to illuminate the frontiers of your ongoing progress. Awareness is the key to breaking the cycle of stress, and encompasses all of the nine steps, while the flame of your hope will grow stronger with your practice of the nine steps. These powerful beacons will always be available to help you and point you in the right direction.

Where To Begin

I recommend starting by reading Part Two: The Nine Natural Steps in its entirety. After this initial reading, you can decide how you will implement the steps in your own life. For example, you may want to choose two steps and begin practicing these first. Once you become familiar and comfortable with your first two steps, start to gradually include more steps until you are practicing all nine in your daily life. Although the steps are numbered one to nine, there is no required order and you are encouraged to begin with the steps to which you are most strongly drawn, with the accompanying advice that I recommend including one of the practical steps in your beginning practice.

People sometimes ask me how to begin the nine steps, telling me that they feel sluggish, run down, and find it hard to take charge. In many cases, an excellent way to begin is to focus on Steps 5, 6, and 7. Ask yourself, how much C.R.A.P. am I eating? And how can I eat Good-Mood Foods instead? And then, how can I introduce a daily walk into my life and begin to be aware of my sleep habits? By focusing on Exercise and Nutrition—especially avoiding C.R.A.P. and seeking out Good-Mood Foods—you also lay the groundwork for better sleep, greater self-awareness, and increased clarity, some of the first keys to wellness. This is also a useful starting point for anyone suffering from a mind condition who is unable to muster the willpower to make the initial changes in the first three steps, for in taking the leap of following Steps 5, 6, and 7 to the best of one's ability, willpower will naturally develop.

This is not to discourage anyone who feels ready to dive right into all nine steps from the beginning. It is for each individual to decide the appropriate program, depending on his or her needs, with the aim of eventually mastering all nine steps in one's life. In any case, I strongly recommend including at least one of the practical steps in your beginning practice. Step 5, Exercise, is a powerful way to begin because it also aids with sleep and, indirectly, nutrition. When people ask me for a suggestion on which step to start with, I invariably advise them to begin practicing Step 5. It is important to begin with one of the Practical Steps, as the benefits become evident early on and begin to precipitate change throughout your life. This creates a foundation upon which the other steps can also develop.

Ultimately, it is the synergy of the nine steps working together that facilitates rapid and lasting transformation; whereas most approaches to health address imbalances in isolation, the nine steps see apparently disparate factors—such as obesity, mind conditions, and addictions—as intricately linked. The ultimate goal, therefore, is to be practicing the steps in harmony, but powerful gains can still be found in commitment to even one or two steps. I recommend beginning in a way that feels natural and then moving on to more when the time is right. As awareness of your lifestyle develops, along with self-awareness, you will make faster progress and eventually be able to naturally incorporate more of the nine steps into your everyday life. In time your symptoms of stress will recede, your neurochemistry will become balanced, your stress response calmed, and you will have completely restyled yourself by mastering stress. You will have taken back control of your life.

Finally, I want to note that the eventual stage of living the nine steps in harmony is not a place of strict discipline. I call this destination the LifeReStyle Solution, and once reached, it is no longer necessary to be practicing all of the steps every day. At this stage, self-awareness and awareness of your lifestyle have developed to a point where you can enjoy different foods and experiences in moderation, without using them as crutches or destructive coping mechanisms. The LifeReStyle process has empowered your mind and body; you have freed yourself of destructive habits; and your awareness of your senses, thoughts, actions, and consequences has developed. Your neurochemistry is balanced and your stress response is activated only occasionally and only when appropriate; you have taken back control of your life and broken the cycle of stress. Having reached this stage, you are then able to let go of the daily practice suggestions of the nine steps and enjoy living in a new way.

Find a pace that is exciting in its challenge, yet not overwhelming. Remember, the Nine Natural Steps are designed to free you of harmful stress, not to create more. They require commitment, but try not to see it as burdensome "work." Enjoy the challenge. You are laying the foundations of your path to mastering stress and thriving.

Valuing yourself allows you
*to live life to its fullest.*_{PH}

Be the change.

Make the difference.

Take one step at a time,

slowly but surely._{PH}

A single thought is like

dropping a pebble into a pond

and watching the ripple effect

*flowing on with awareness.*_{PH}

PART TWO

The Nine Natural Steps

Nine Natural Steps

STEP 1

TAKE CHARGE

Only the wisest and the stupidest
of men never change.
Confucius

Are you in charge of your life?

The key to beating stress is in making the simple decision to do so. It is the decision to take charge of your life and reclaim your power that opens the way to change. All the other steps follow naturally from this point.

The first step in breaking the cycle of stress is a shift of your mind-set to a place where you recognize, first, that you experience stress and, second, that the cause of this stress is your accumulated habits: the "old you." Your commitment to implementing change in your life is the gateway to progress. If you are suffering from serious stress-related consequences, then this is the key to freeing yourself and reclaiming your power. If you are not suffering from stress-related illnesses, then this is an opportunity to prevent such conditions from arising and to beat stress in your life. In either case, your commitment to change is the key to discovering true contentment and joy.

You're worth it

You must realize that a full life, free of harmful stress, is your birthright. Many of us have difficulty loving ourselves, and so we allow ourselves to get dragged into a disharmonious way of life. This compromises our physical and mental health. The simple truth is that if we valued our well-being to the degree that it deserves, we would approach our lives very differently. Realize that as a human being you deserve love, and you deserve love from yourself. Understand that valuing your well-being, and living your life free of stress and with contentment, is an act of love. It is what you deserve. Furthermore, know that it *is* possible; you can achieve this, and you can change your life. There were periods during my experiences with severe depression and bipolar disorder that were unbearably demoralizing and dark, when hope was entirely absent. And yet I have found, and we have all seen at different times, that the potential for change in people's lives is real. It is possible for every single one of us.

Accepting the need for change

The beginning of change for the better in your life is the awareness that something *must* change. This awareness that unnecessary stress exists and is taking a toll on your life leads to the next logical step, which is deciding what to do about it. It is essential to accept that it is the "old you" that is the cause of stress or illness. Your old way of doing things is the reason that harmful stress or illness exists. Therefore, it is necessary to be proactive about changing your life, allowing yourself to change, and breaking destructive habits. Only you can do this.

*Life is never fair; life is what you make it.*_{PH}

By understanding that stress is the result of your reaction to challenges in your life, the following nine steps can be implemented to undo destructive habits and strengthen the mind and body. The new, healthy, and balanced life that you are building is its own reward.

Taking the first step of accepting the need for change and being proactive about making that change can present challenges. In many cases, this decision can feel more like a giant leap instead of a step. It can be a choice that you keep returning to time and again, renewing and strengthening your commitment. In my experience with people suffering from stress-related conditions, I've often noticed a strong sense of denial and a failure to realize that we have the opportunity to change our lives. We can take charge of our own health and peace of mind. It is up to us to exercise our free will.

Right now, at this very moment, take stock of where you are. Consider your mind and body and what they are telling you. Are you sleeping well? Do you spend a lot of time worrying? Do you experience anxiety or suffer from physical tension or illnesses? If you feel stressed, the body is sending you a message that something is out of balance and that something needs to change. By heeding this warning, you can change your life for the better. Allow any symptoms of stress to be your barometer of wellness. Your present lifestyle is of your own creation; if you are unhappy in any way, take the first step and begin to restyle your life.

It's never ever too late

to be wise.

Daniel Defoe, *Robinson Crusoe*

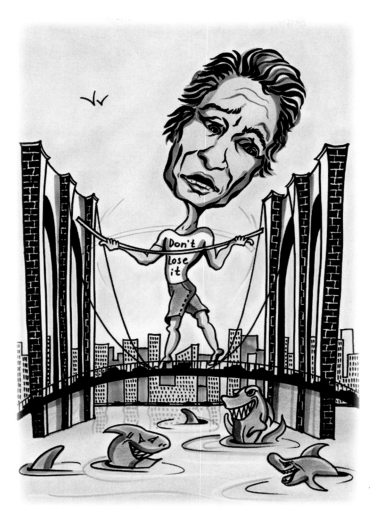

Don't lose it. Prevention is the key.

Take responsibility for your own life.
If you want to see a change for the better,
you have to take things into your own hands.
Clint Eastwood

Be proactive

Having acknowledged the need for change, it becomes your responsibility to take charge of your life. Only you know, deep down, what is best for you. While it is important to be open to advice from others, what matters most is that you take full responsibility for your life and any changes you need to make, which will take shape as you put the nine steps into practice. It is necessary to be proactive in changing your way of life, thus turning your life around if you are already in the grip of stress-related illness or, if you have not been seriously affected by stress, preventing stress-related conditions and building longevity. It's time to rebuild yourself.

The habits that brought you to your present situation have evolved over time. The nine steps are about creating new patterns to replace old habits that have created your current situation. Many people feel stuck at first, and they may make excuses or refuse to find the necessary time each day to effect true change. However, by committing time each day to implementing the nine steps, your life will begin to shift.

Be proactive, fortify and empower yourself,
*and say No to stress.*_{PH}

Making time

Your time is precious. This is a huge issue and usually the first obstacle to overcome in reclaiming one's power. We are often kept to a very tough schedule; it's easy to be overwhelmed and lose control. I've had a great deal of experience with the challenge of making time for balanced living, and in the past I have often fallen victim to my tendency to give more of my time and energy than I could realistically spare, leaving me exhausted and unable to find time for what was most important to me. In failing to take charge of my life, I experienced a great deal of stress, which in turn disrupted my neurochemical balance. I have found that it is essential to take control and dedicate a portion of each day to maintaining one's body and mind.

Putting the nine steps into practice may call for reprioritizing your routine. You may need to start your days a little earlier, or set aside time at night for the practices that will break habits and strengthen the new you. Your usual schedule will likely need to be modified, and some of your existing leisure time may need to be devoted to the positive changes you are making in your life. This can sometimes present difficulties, especially when your new routines affect friends and family members, and it can be a challenge to your progress if people find the new you that is emerging threatening to the status quo. However, the nine steps also eliminate a lot of time-consuming inefficiency, and in the end this may allow more true, quality time with friends, family, and the activities that you enjoy most. **The LifeReStyle solution is designed for people on the go with restricted time and as such it offers maximum benefit for minimum time and effort.**

*No one knows you better than you do.*_{PH}

It's not just that you deserve change yourself, but also that your loved ones, too, will ultimately benefit from your balance and health. Think of the people in your life and how heartbroken they might be if you gave up on yourself or became ill from stress: taking charge of your life isn't just done for your own sake, but for the sake of others, too.

In making the necessary time to put the nine steps into practice, you will discover that this is *your* time to maintain and reinforce your personal well-being. Putting time aside for your own health and development enhances all the other activities in your life; it allows you to more fully enjoy being with family, friends, in the workplace, and in recreation as you are able to live with greater freedom from stress. In time you will be far more productive, functioning at a higher level with increased contentment, laughter, and joy. You will not only survive the stress pandemic, but thrive.

At first, time schedule adjustments, reprioritization, and departure from your former lifestyle may leave you feeling tired or disoriented. This is perfectly normal during a period of transition. If you think of a glass of murky water into which clear water is poured, it takes time for the murky water to be displaced and for the vessel to become completely clear. This is a useful analogy for understanding the process of change in our own lives. The changes in your life can't normally happen overnight, but you will quickly begin to see and feel increasing benefits from your efforts.

*Prevention is the key.*_{PH}

Renew your commitment

Developing a new lifestyle is bound to be met with obstacles and disappointments from time to time. Expect that you will encounter challenges and that you won't always perform perfectly in implementing the nine steps. Like a child learning to walk, you must realize that you will inevitably fall over at times. Don't let this dampen your enthusiasm; let it fuel your focus even more. Whenever you stumble, brush yourself off and get up again, keeping your vision set on the well-being that you deserve. Use every disappointment and every so-called "failure" as an opportunity to renew your commitment to beating stress and living fully.

*Take charge and stay in charge.*_{PH}

Taking Charge: Daniel's Story

I would like to share three stories of people who took the first step and quickly turned their lives around. While traveling through Boston during a book tour, I met a middle-aged man named Daniel who was well-spoken, well-educated, and addicted to cocaine. His health was suffering, he experienced severe sleeping issues due to vivid nightmares, and he was unable to cope with the increasing stress of his complicated life. I explained to him in depth the nine steps, gave him some affirmations that I felt were well-suited to his situation, and wished him the best.

A few months later I received an email from Daniel

expressing his gratitude and excitement for the new life he had begun. He had read this book soon after our meeting and had decided to throw himself headlong into the nine steps. He had quit cocaine, recovered his health, found balance in his life, and experienced much greater self-esteem. He reported that his nightmares had ceased and that he felt lighter and happier.

Taking Charge: Lucy's Story

This second story I share to illustrate how stress can affect people of any age. I met a lady in Chicago named Sophie whose five-year-old granddaughter Lucy had recently been diagnosed with bipolar disorder. Doctors had wanted to prescribe medication for Lucy; Sophie was beside herself in light of the situation and unsure of what she could do. With Lucy's single mother being a busy media executive, it was Sophie who spent the most time taking care of the young girl. She shared with me her granddaughter's medical history and her present daily routine and asked for some practical suggestions.

I thought it unfortunate that Lucy had been diagnosed with such a severe condition at such a young age, because from what I was told, it seemed that the outbursts that she was demonstrating should first be addressed with a more appropriate daily routine and an attempt to introduce more stability and affection into Lucy's life. I told Sophie to take Lucy for a brisk walk each morning for whatever amount of time felt right for such a young person to ensure she was getting some physical activity before school; afterward, she should make a small glass of fresh vegetable juice for her granddaughter and serve a healthy breakfast of natural oatmeal or muesli—with no additives—

and fresh fruit. I advised her to pack a nutritious lunch and to encourage Lucy to drink room temperature water first thing in the morning and throughout the day. C.R.A.P. was to be completely removed from Lucy's diet (see Step 6) and I suggested closely monitoring her intake of television and keeping it to a minimum while avoiding anything that could be stimulating or stressful for Lucy for an hour before her bedtime. Instead, as bedtime neared, I advised Sophie to tell her stories that expressed how grateful she was for her granddaughter, which were a form of affirmation that would comfort and calm Lucy. I told her to ensure that Lucy received plenty of hugs and kisses and I suggested rubbing Lucy's tummy in a circular motion as she was preparing for sleep, while stroking her hair and forehead to calm her and let her know how loved she was.

To Sophie's great credit, she took the bull by the horns and put everything into practice. She phoned me within in a few weeks overflowing with joy to tell me that her granddaughter was completely transformed. She thought the shift was amazing. I responded that it did seem amazing, but that it's really just the power of natural healing; it was nature simply working its magic. But, of course, this could never have happened were it not for Sophie taking charge of the situation and committing to making sweeping changes in her granddaughter's routine, given that Lucy was too young to make those changes herself.

Taking Charge: Maggie's Story

The final story involves a woman from New York named Maggie who came to me saying that she didn't have the will power to improve her life. She told me that she started her day at eleven a.m. and that there was nothing she could do to make herself feel good. "This is who I am," she insisted with frustration and despair. "I'm depressed and I have been this way for years. My parents and siblings are obese. I'm obese. I'm lonely, my life is physically and emotionally painful, and one of the few things I like to do is drink alcohol."

My answer was that there is a natural magic potion, but that she had to reach for it herself. I could help guide her by giving her the tools, road map, and compass, but the effort had to come from within her. If she would just give it a chance, she might be surprised by how she could heal. "This is all about you, Maggie," I told her. "You have the free will to take back control."

Of course, she had probably already tried in some way, perhaps more than once, to turn her life around but been met with failure. So I continued, "Think of yourself as having a broken leg, let's say with multiple fractures. It may take time for the natural healing process to run its course, and the initiation and speed of that process will depend on what actions you take. You can't try to walk around or run too early in the healing process. You have to commit to allowing nature to work its magic, and then respect the process."

I could see her thinking carefully about what I had said and then I added a further analogy. "Don't get overwhelmed by this process. Do you drive a car?" She nodded. "Before stepping into it, do you mentally review all of the lessons and experiences you went through as a teenager in order to be able to first drive a car?" She indicated that she did not. "When you did first learn to drive, did you do it by seeing the whole process laid out in print, agonizing over all the hard work you would need to do over time and the stages through which you would have to pass in order to be a good driver?" She smiled. "No, of course you didn't. Someone who had learned years before and had plenty of experience driving cars took you through the steps and equipped you with everything you needed in order to be a competent driver. Hopefully it was a fun, exciting, sometimes scary process. But if you had begun by obsessing over what was to come, perhaps you never would have made it out of the parking lot. This process is no different. This book is your teacher, and you only need to take one step at a time. Trust that committing to the process will enable the natural healing process to take you where you need to go."

I suggested that Maggie start with one step in order to build her confidence and willpower. If she couldn't start her day until eleven a.m., then fine, at eleven a.m. take a walk for forty to sixty minutes in the sun, immersed in nature if possible. She thought seriously about all that I had said and, after some time, told me that she wanted to restyle her life. From that simple beginning of a daily walk, Maggie made huge strides in her journey. She phoned me several months later to inform me that she had gradually adopted one step after another, never rushing, never losing hope, but just patiently re-building her life and letting nature steadily support her in her healing. She told me that she had become a mostly confident and happy person who no longer allowed the world to bully her. She started her day at six a.m. with her brisk morning walk and, lately, had received numerous compliments from friends and acquaintances who could not quite believe that this was actually Maggie.

All three of these accounts demonstrate how decisively

things can turn around once we fully commit to the first step and let the rest follow from there. Take the first step: resolve to take charge of your life.

> *If you are distressed by anything external,*
> *The pain is not due to the thing itself*
> *but to your estimate of it;*
> *and this you have the power*
> *to revoke at any moment.*
> Marcus Aurelius

SUMMARY

STEP 1 : Take Charge

- Know that you deserve well-being and balance.
- Accept the need for change—recognize that the "old you" has caused stress.
- Take charge—take responsibility for making changes and implementing the nine steps of the LifeReStyle Process.
- Be aware of any symptoms of stress arising in your life.
- Make time each day for putting the nine steps into practice.
- Renew your commitment every time you fall. Take charge and stay in charge.

Questions to ask yourself:

- How do I create stress in my life?
- How do I respond to challenges and stressful situations?
- How do I maintain my body and mind to be able to withstand stress?
- Am I aware of where I am in my life right now?
- Am I aware of any symptoms and dangers of stress in my body and mind?
- How do I use my time? Am I using my time efficiently so I can put these changes into action?
- Am I fortifying and empowering myself?

Life is full of temptations,

controlling and challenging you with fear and greed;

breaking the cycle of bad habits

*requires great perseverance and courage.*_{PH}

KICK YOUR BAD HABITS

Every form of addiction is bad,
no matter whether the narcotic be
alcohol or morphine or idealism.
Carl Jung

Are your bad habits controlling your lifestyle?

The Nine Natural Steps are, at a basic level, about identifying and changing habits. Many of our habitual coping mechanisms for dealing with stress are destructive or harmful, and this is the area to which we now turn our attention.

Most of us develop certain habits as coping mechanisms and outlets for stress. To beat stress, it is essential to overcome destructive coping mechanisms so that you can deal with stress directly. You can then become more aware of the underlying cause of your stress, whether it's your response to some challenge, or choices you make that are at odds with your innermost feelings. This enables you to address issues directly, rather than allowing them to fester by avoiding the root cause through some form of distraction.

Identify your destructive coping mechanisms

A destructive coping mechanism could accurately be looked upon as a type of addiction. Like most habits, destructive coping mechanisms have an addictive quality to them; we feel some degree of compulsion toward them, and we experience some level of difficulty in resisting them. We also tend to use a destructive coping mechanism as a distraction, a crutch that we lean on as a way of avoiding stress. These activities, then, are no longer true choices that we make but rather are unconscious habits that often prevent us from dealing directly with stress and are therefore harmful to our well-being.

Addictions can take many forms, both obvious and subtle. Some are clearly harmful, such as reliance on alcohol, prescription or recreational drugs, gambling, smoking, or dysfunctional eating. Almost anything can become an addiction, though, from watching TV to exercise, computer use, work, or even socializing. While these may not immediately appear to be destructive, make no mistake that on a very real level they encroach on your time, sap your attention, and prevent you from living fully. Even something as natural and enjoyable as sex can become an addiction and exhibit these characteristics. These habits do not generate any true joy but instead are a source of obsession that constantly needs to be satisfied. Finally, coping mechanisms mask the true stress you are experiencing in your life, preventing you from dealing with the source of the problem. This stress can grow and become truly harmful if it is left unchecked.

*Addictions and habits are learned, not genetic.*_{PH}

After speaking with many people who live with serious addictions, I have found that most addictions form gradually over time. Some people begin experimenting with drugs, but when the impact of the drug starts to wane, they turn to stronger drugs or more frequent encounters. I've noticed the same thing with alcohol, where a person may make a habit of enjoying a glass of wine each night, but eventually the amount creeps up until daily intake becomes a cause for concern. After my breakdown, I reviewed my own life and realized that I had many addictions, though I would never have recognized these as "addictions" or "destructive coping mechanisms" until I examined my behavior closely. Even a supposedly easily identifiable one, such as alcohol, wasn't an obvious addiction, because I wouldn't have qualified as an "alcoholic."

However, in making an honest assessment, I had to admit that my wife and I were, at times, drinking a bottle of wine with dinner every night, and that this was fueled largely by my growing anxiety and unhappiness. Other behaviors may have seemed more innocent, but still, they were a reaction to my stress levels. My cravings for large bowls of popcorn or multiple packets of cookies at night while watching movies in bed were not conscious choices for normal portions but rather mindless, compulsive eating where I would consume the snack of the moment, pursuing temporary escape from the challenges of my life. Later I was to understand that I had become addicted to the *dopamine high* of junk food. What was more, my neurochemistry developed a greater tolerance for junk food and, as with all addictions, increasing amounts of the substance were gradually required to induce a dopamine high. Later, I had to be aware of this so that I didn't allow my dopamine reward system to be "hijacked" by an artificial stimulant.

Dopamine is a neurochemical that helps control the brain's reward and pleasure centers. It is crucial for learning adaptive behaviors, however addictive habits or substances exploit this normal mechanism by flooding the brain with dopamine. Such behaviors light up the brain's pleasure circuitry, often bringing a burst of euphoria. We tend to want to maximize pleasure; we tend to do things that bring more of it. We also tend to chase after pleasure when it subsides, hoping to recreate the same level of pleasure we have experienced in the past. The word "addiction" is derived from a Latin term for "enslaved by" or "bound to." Anyone who has struggled with an addiction can understand why. In a person who becomes addicted, brain receptors become overwhelmed. The brain responds by producing less dopamine or eliminating dopamine receptors, effectively dampening the effect of future floods of dopamine. As a result, people build up a tolerance to such habits and the dopamine produced has less impact on the brain's reward center. An individual then has to take more of a substance or engage more in a particular behavior in order to obtain the same dopamine "high."

*Is your dopamine being hijacked?*PH

Exercise Strict Moderation

Moderation is a concept that's often difficult for us to grasp. We have to understand that tolerances build and, though we often feel that we aren't leaning on destructive coping mechanisms, we may often be flirting with danger. As our dopamine system is hijacked we build tolerance for the objects of our addictions and we can lose control long before we know it. The journey back to freedom and balance can be harsh and it can be a difficult battle to win. This is why it's important to take stock of where you are now and begin to examine your coping mechanisms.

In thinking about addictions, it's useful to remember the multitude of public personalities who have succumbed to addictions, such as Elvis Presley, Michael Jackson, Karen Carpenter, and Whitney Houston to name a few. From some perspectives, it may appear that these people had everything. Why then would they give up on life?

*Let not your passion become your source of stress.*PH

Even though these individuals' lives were dedicated to following their passion and what they enjoyed most, what was initially a source of enjoyment eventually became a source of great pressure. In attempting to deal with this pressure, they turned to very harmful coping mechanisms.

Clearly, if you struggle with addictions of any kind, you are not alone in your struggle, and the accumulation of wealth or status clearly does not render us immune to such challenges. Though we might think that our lives are not what we want them to be, even those who seem to have everything still face the same basic struggles as us all. Such examples demonstrate the slippery slope of addiction; we may think that we are getting something, that our destructive coping mechanisms are helping us, but this is not the reality. I have met so many people who became victims of their addictions. They tell me how they lost everything and how much they wish they had had the clarity to stop before they lost control. In many ways an addiction is like quicksand: often by the time you become aware of an addiction, it can be too late. Where is the tipping point?

Practice moderation. Don't allow
*your dopamine to be hijacked.*_{PH}

Mental and emotional patterns that have an addictive quality are equally as important to address, though they may be harder to recognize in ourselves. This is a key role for an objective, wise outsider. Whether that be a trusted friend, family member, doctor, or therapist, someone both caring and impartial can help bring to light destructive psychological tendencies so that they can be dealt with. Until we are aware of our addictions, we are slaves to them, and we will continue to sabotage ourselves and our progress. While in the Menninger Clinic, I became aware of some of my own psychological addictions, such as the way I approached my work and the building of my business or my unhealthy need to care for others more than I cared for myself, which resulted in my often feeling like a martyr. I also understood that I'd been working at a manic pace and in an addictive mode, often taking my briefcase home and working late nights in my study, then working on Saturdays and Sundays. It was clear that my behaviors had become excessive.

Start by observing where and how you spend your time.

Consider the activities you turn to when you are stressed or uncomfortable. Ask yourself if the way you engage in these activities has an addictive or habitual pattern to it and if you are letting destructive behavior control your life. If you discover certain activities or psychological patterns that are destructive or feel more "addictive" or like a "release" than they do joyful, then make it your goal to gradually free yourself from these addictions. The Nine Natural Steps will help you to do this.

Overcoming addictions

The key to freeing yourself from any destructive coping mechanism or addiction lies in gradually decreasing your reliance until you no longer require any release or stimulation from it. When I initially confronted my addictions, I decided that I did not want to take the approach of organizations such as Alcoholics Anonymous, which advocated completely eradicating an object from one's life. I realized that if I eliminated 100 percent of everything I was addicted to, there wouldn't be much left. Many of my activities had become imbued with an addictive quality, and I resolved to regain control of all these valuable elements in my life instead of using them as coping mechanisms. Eventually, as I became more balanced, my neurochemistry was restored and my addictions were no longer in control; I was. In time, I could then learn to enjoy these elements in my life while maintaining a sense of strict moderation. (There are, however, many addictions that must be eliminated from one's life for good, such as serious addictions to alcohol and drugs, which can be seen to clearly harm one's body and mind even in small doses.)

After you have identified your destructive coping mechanisms, choose one to focus on to begin with, and start monitoring your reliance on it. Going back to Step 1, the most important part of overcoming addiction is your decision and commitment to doing so. Once you have resolved that your well-being is more important than any fleeting release or pleasure you receive from the addiction, you can gradually decrease your reliance on the object every week. Continue to decrease your dependence on the pattern, monitoring it weekly, until you no longer crave the addiction. Continue this reduction process with as many destructive coping mechanisms you can let go of at once. Recognize that some will be relatively easy to overcome, while others will present bigger challenges. It is perseverance that will see you through in the end. It is also important to understand that stress exacerbates our destructive tendencies as we seek escape. For example, stress results in elevated levels of the hunger-inducing hormone ghrelin; it's not difficult to see how this relationship plays into the use of food as a means of avoiding dealing with stress.

*Once you recognize that the "old you" is what made you unwell, you can take ownership of your old behavior and free yourself from being a victim.*PH

Freeing yourself from habits gradually is often much more effective than going cold-turkey. I saw how difficult it was to give up my own coping mechanisms, and I found I didn't have the willpower to say, "Starting tomorrow, I am no longer eating dessert or cookies." It simply didn't work for me. Instead, I monitored my reliance on the habit in question and would, for example, ask for a smaller piece of dessert. I continued decreasing the size until I could then say no to dessert altogether. At times I found myself taking extra measures to ensure that I wouldn't be tempted—for example, asking other members of the family not to eat certain foods in front of me or asking them to hide certain foods. This would help to ensure that I wouldn't be triggered and tempted to undo the progress I was making toward beating my addictions to alcohol and food.

It is important to remember that things will not always go smoothly and that you will encounter setbacks, perhaps even resorting to your old ways. Write down each success or disappointment every day so that you are aware of your progress and never fooling yourself. Keep a diary of your progress and take stock of your wins and losses with each coping mechanism. Since habits are generally formed over a thirty-day period, when you can complete a full thirty-day period of independence from an addiction, you can consider yourself successful in that particular battle. Your cravings will then readjust and balance, and you will grow in willpower, energy, and focus, as you free yourself from self-destructive habits.

If for any reason you give in to an addiction prior to the completion of thirty days, the count would begin again at day one. For example, if you feel dependent on alcohol to some degree—major or minor—and you are working on freeing yourself of this dependency, but end up having a glass of wine on day twenty-four, then a new count of thirty days would need to begin at that point.

We often deal with stress through coping mechanisms, some of which are more destructive and addictive than others. It's important to address those that are destructive, but ultimately all coping mechanisms become secondary to our process of dealing with stress and we are able to meet stress head-on. You might still use benign coping mechanisms, but the nine steps will eventually enable you to fortify yourself against stress and master it so that you are no longer reliant on coping mechanisms. This is being able to live freely. We all reach for various tools at different times to deal with stress, but we are often unaware of the best way to use them or we reach for the wrong tools. The nine steps identify the instruments that you need to break the cycle of stress; the nine steps become your new toolbox.

Destructive coping mechanisms are an artificial way of combating stress. Confronting them is one of the most powerful things you can do. Remember that it will take time, but that by identifying your addictions and deciding to overcome them, you have already begun the process. As you put the other steps in this book into practice, they will also support you in beating your addictions. All of the nine steps are interdependent, reinforcing one another in supporting your well-being, strength, and freedom from stress.

*The mind is constantly seeking and craving satisfaction, desiring to have its thoughts fulfilled.*PH

Kicking Your Bad Habits: Betty's Story

I find it interesting to note two dynamics relating to coping mechanisms that I've seen demonstrated in many people's lives. The first is that people develop destructive coping mechanisms as a result of stress. The second, related dynamic is that destructive coping mechanisms usually can't be addressed solely on their own level; they are deeply rooted in underlying stress and therefore lasting change only comes when the whole person is attended to, rather than simply focusing on one behavior pattern that is an outward manifestation of a deeper dynamic. Betty's story illustrates both of these points in simple ways.

Betty came to me while I was speaking in Washington, DC, and told me she was in constant pain. She was a single mother of two in her early forties working in middle management. Her husband had abandoned her and her children for a younger woman a number of years ago. Betty was taking antidepressants and sleep medication, and her greatest fear was of becoming seriously ill and not being able to provide for her children. She was worried about her position at work and felt that she had recently been overlooked for a promotion. I asked her how she felt about herself and she responded that she loved her children, but that whenever she looked in the mirror she felt unhappy.

"What do you do when you're unhappy or stressed?" I asked her.

"I like my desserts and I like my wine," she said, adding that New Zealand made some of her favorite bottles of sauvignon blanc and chardonnay.

Betty had not always been overweight, but over time she

had increasingly turned to comfort food to deal with her pain, eventually putting on excess weight. She couldn't stop herself and had developed an addiction not only to an unhealthy relationship with comfort food, but also to yo-yo dieting. She would frequently start a new diet, lose some weight, and then put it all back on soon after.

I told Betty that there were a few things she needed to acknowledge and fully understand. First, she needed to face the fact that there was unhappiness and stress that she was attempting to escape through food and alcohol. I explained to her the relationship between food, addiction, and neuro-chemical balance. These factors had created the pattern of turning to food and alcohol as a destructive coping mechanism. Next, I told Betty that trying to control her weight simply by dieting would not work. Her pattern involved multiple levels of habits and lifestyle, and she therefore needed to address those multiple levels. As you may notice with other stories in this book, while a problem may manifest on one level—such as diet, exercise, relationships—it's really the whole person that needs to be addressed. This is why using the nine steps to address the varied problems that people suffer from usually involves attending to the practical elements of nutrition, exercise, and sleep, as well as the more internal dynamics outlined in these earlier steps.

I told Betty that the root cause of her suffering was stress; this was causing her to make poor lifestyle decisions which, in turn, generated more stress. She needed to restyle and fortify herself and I suggested she begin by implementing Steps 5 (Exercise) and 6 (Nutrition). Specifically, if she made a concerted effort to cut down on the C.R.A.P. in her diet, as outlined in Step 6, while simultaneously introducing the brisk morning walk outlined in Step 5 into her routine, the two steps would work together to enable her to steadily change her ways. These would be of great assistance in addressing her major problem, her destructive coping mechanisms (Step 2); without incorporating the other steps, however, she would be unlikely to gather the momentum and willpower to shift her destructive behaviors. With the support of all three of these steps working in synergy, she would build the ability to face the root stress and unhappiness that was causing her imbalances in the first place and, as she continued on her journey with the nine steps, she would eventually be able to take greater control of her life and steadily improve her situation.

I am delighted to report that after some time Betty got in touch with me to share her excitement at how she had transformed her life. While she still had further to go, she felt her life was turning around. She was no longer taking sleeping tablets; she had lost weight; and with the strict guidance of her psychiatrist, her reliance on antidepressants had been greatly reduced. In addition, she had received a promotion and, for the first time in years, Betty was feeling good about the future. Her sense of awareness was developing and she felt excited about what lay ahead as she continued to reshape her life.

> *It is easier to prevent bad habits*
> *than to break them.*
> Benjamin Franklin

The important thing is this,

to be able at any moment to sacrifice what we are

for what we could become.

Charles du Bois

SUMMARY

STEP 2 : Kick Your Bad Habits

- Observe how you spend your time, noticing if certain patterns feel more "addictive," or like a "release," than enjoyable.
- Consider whether or not these patterns are harmful to your well-being or limit your true enjoyment of life.
- Resolve to overcome your destructive coping mechanisms, beginning with one at a time, and taking on what you can comfortably manage as you free yourself from harmful habits. Free yourself from the dopamine hijack of addictive patterns and destructive coping mechanisms.
- Gradually decrease your dependence on each addictive pattern, monitoring your daily progress in writing.
- Continue monitoring the addiction until you have completed a thirty-day period of total independence from the pattern.
- Recognize that beating addictions takes time and can be challenging and that your practice of all of the nine steps will assist in freeing you from destructive coping mechanisms.

Questions to ask yourself:

- How reliant am I on my habits?
- Are there patterns I turn to when I'm stressed?
- If so, are these activities a crutch, and am I using them to avoid or mask stress?
- Am I enjoying things in moderation, or am I being excessive?
- How do these habits affect my life and well-being?
- Am I fortifying and empowering myself?
- Am I breaking my bad habits following the 30 day liferestyle process?

It is not what we do,

but also what we do not do,

for which we are accountable.

Molière

(Jean-Baptiste Poquelin)

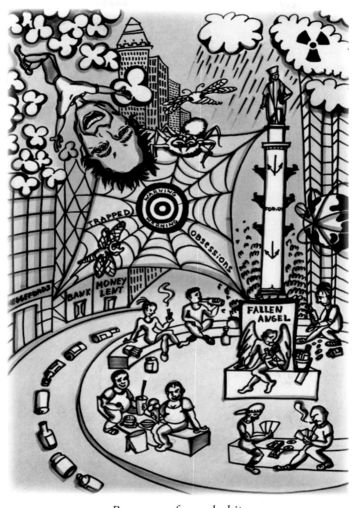

Be aware of your habits.

Learn to say No.

Follow your innermost feelings.

No one knows you

*better than yourself.*_{PH}

∼∾∾e

STEP 3

LEARN TO SAY NO

No one saves us but ourselves. No one can and no one may. We ourselves must walk the path.
Siddhartha Gautama

We live in a world that has become a bit of a bullying place. What are you doing about it?

To break the cycle of stress, we need to be true to ourselves. Whenever we are not true to ourselves, we create disharmony that is painful or that gradually festers and saps our life of joy, building resentment and disturbing our piece of mind. By learning to say No to whatever is detrimental to your well-being and instead following your innermost feelings, you will begin to experience a strong sense of contentment in your life and in the decisions you make. Even when inevitable bad times or challenges arise, you will be able to weather those storms with inner strength.

Undesirable situations in our lives are often the result of failing to listen to our innermost feelings. This can lead us to overcommit ourselves, overpush ourselves, or get involved in something that is not what we truly want. By doing so, we create disharmony within, that activates the stress response and disrupts our neurochemistry. In exercising free will to say and do what we desire, as long as we're not hurting ourselves or others, we become more centered and balanced. This results in an abiding sense of contentment in the knowledge that, even when some decisions are difficult, we've done what we felt we had to do.

As with every other recommended change in this book, Step 3 will challenge you. It will challenge you to summon the courage to know your innermost feelings and follow them more and more each day, knowing that in prioritizing this commitment, you are prioritizing your well-being.

*The world has become a bit of a bullying place.*PH

Learning to say No

No one else knows our thoughts and feelings with certainty, so it is up to us to set our own boundaries, being firm about what we can or can't do. It is so easy in this world to take on too many commitments. We often feel obligated to people and projects that we know are only taking time that we can't really spare. This can build up resentment and anger. You need to be able to say No—or at least No for the moment, or "not now," in order to give yourself time to think things over—and do what's right for yourself in order to preserve the person you are. If you don't learn to say No, your stress levels will rise as you live in disharmony with your true desires and in disharmony with the amount of time and energy you truly have. In finding the courage to decline obligations and demands that you know you can't meet, you also allow people to know the true you and your true wishes. This is not selfishness in the negative sense of the word; it is honesty. No matter what reasoning people give us as to why we should say Yes to their wishes or demands, it is for us to be strong, stand our ground, and communicate how we truly feel and what we are truly capable of.

In my own experience, I realized at one time that I wasn't even aware of what my own true feelings were on a lot of matters. I had become so accustomed to wanting to please others, especially those I cared about, that I found it very difficult to say No or to tell the truth about what I thought. I had to train myself, which took time. During this period of readjustment, I would at times agree to something that I later wished I hadn't, or vice versa. It was a process of reprogramming and relearning how to set boundaries. Denying your true feelings due to fear of the response or because you are eager to please will only cause resentment in the long run as your discontent with a situation accumulates. I came to acknowledge that there was a huge amount of stress tied up in my attempts to please those around me. My desire to keep everyone happy placed a huge strain on my time and energy. In the end, I realized that more than anything, I had betrayed myself and could blame no one else but myself.

Saying No is one of the most important ingredients in a life filled with peace of mind and contentment. This is not a No rooted in cynicism or emotional withdrawal; with the ability to say No comes balance and healthy boundaries. Despite the benefits of this universally understood word, many of us have a hard time saying it for fear of upsetting someone else, and we may end up feeling burdened, resentful, and even victimized. Ironically, we forget that we were the ones who said Yes in the first place.

We often wear an emotional mask to hide our feelings. It is like the saying "many faces we wear". Sometimes its good to stop for a moment and say No, and be true to yourself. It may be very difficult to do, but ultimately you can look in the mirror and know the face you chose to show the world is how you feel in your heart. A true reflection of yourself!

*Don't be a martyr or a puppet; just be yourself.*PH

Practice saying No to commitments, obligations, and requests from others that you don't truly believe in or that you know won't serve you well in the long run. In more faithfully following your true desires and goals, you will begin to have more time and energy for the people and activities that are of real value to you. This will eliminate some of the unnecessary demands on your time and energy that only generate stress. Whether it's a boss, a spouse, friends, or family, people's wishes are not always in line with our own. We must be honest when we are unable to meet those wishes or demands, not only for the sake of our own health but also to serve our true goals and desires and to allow others to know who we really are. Although this may not always be comfortable and may present a variety of challenges, especially for those who are more sensitive and thus more susceptible to emotional stress, it is an important component of reclaiming the power that is your birthright.

Once, after a talk I gave in Seattle, I met a lady named Jenny who appeared to "have it all." What she shared with me, however, was that for as long as she could remember she had been bullied by her older sister, Allison. Jenny felt completely unable to say no to her sister and she asked for advice on how to deal with the situation.

I told Jenny that the most important thing was that, whatever she does, she feels that she has done her best. She needed to be true to herself. The situation wasn't about her sister; it was about Jenny's ability to set boundaries. I advised Jenny to apply the steps in the book as well as she could, as this would build her strength in being able to handle these stressful situations. The time would soon come when she would need to sit down with her sister, face to face, and be honest with her about the situation, despite the very real feelings of discomfort that would likely arise. I suggested using a specific affirmation, such as "I, Jenny, have the strength, courage, and wisdom to communicate honestly with my sister and stand up for myself." Jenny asked what would happen if her sister didn't listen and respect her wishes, and I said that as difficult as it may be, she would then have to consider putting some space between her and her sister in order to move forward with her life. As sad as it is, we sometimes must be honest about a particular relationship that is harming us and decide to take action so that we can either claim our space from the relationship, or so it can grow into a truly loving and supportive relationship,

Learn to follow your innermost feelings

Just as important as the art of saying No is knowing when to say Yes. Both responses are part of the same development process, which is learning to discern and communicate your innermost feelings. We are constantly being told what our feelings should be—and how we should respond—through our upbringing and family or through culture, environment, and advertising. For example, you may believe that a promotion at work is the key to more happiness, only to find that after all the hard work required to earn the promotion, the promotion swallows more of your precious time and creates too much pressure in your life. This is not to say that you shouldn't work for a promotion or that you shouldn't want to grow in your work, but it is important to be aware, consult your inner voice, and be clear about what you actually want.

*Willpower has as much to do with saying No to the bad things in life as it does with passionately saying Yes to the good things.*_{PH}

In learning to follow your innermost feelings, there will be times when you will not know immediately what you truly want. It will be necessary to pause and reflect for a moment, deeply considering the decision you're about to make. Sometimes it will require time and reflection, and it also requires training and practice. The true test of that practice is if you have a sense of contentment and are free of stress, anger, and resentment surrounding a particular decision. It is useful to keep track of decisions you make, noting differences between quick choices, carefully considered ones, and whether you chose Yes or No. Look back later on to evaluate how earlier decisions turned out, seeing if there is anything to learn about how the decisions were made. Have the courage to follow through on how you feel, making choices that are true to the person you really are. In this way you will live in greater harmony with your true self, minimizing the amount of stress you experience from misplaced time and energy and increasing the level of contentment and joy you experience in your life.

From time to time you may find yourself looking back and wishing you had chosen differently in a decision. Maybe you entered a career you didn't really want or married someone who wasn't right for you or took on more responsibility as you tried to get a bigger home, and now you find that these decisions haven't brought you the happiness you expected. There are no guarantees in life, but wherever you are, you can begin living in closer alignment with your innermost feelings starting today, knowing that you can't be sure of what will happen, but at least you did your best. That is where the courage lies.

Avoid unnecessary pain
of the mind and the body;
sometimes the pain man inflicts on himself
is far more terrifying
*than what nature inflicts on man.*_{PH}

Learning to say No is challenging at first.

The more you can say it,

*the stronger you will become.*_{PH}

SUMMARY

STEP 3 : Learn to Say No

- Learn to say No to demands and requests that are not in line with your true desires. Don't commit to obligations that you do not have the necessary time and energy for.
- Learn to discern your innermost feelings.
- Record decisions that you've made and how you made them so you can learn from their outcomes at a later date and compare similar situations in the future.
- Practice following your innermost feelings so that, regardless of whether things work out the way you want them to, you know that you have done your best and have been true to yourself.

Questions to ask yourself:

- Am I agreeing to something, taking on a commitment, or prioritizing someone else's wishes, while not truly wanting to?
- Do I have the necessary time and energy to devote to commitments that I don't feel strongly about, or are they causing substantial and unnecessary stress in my life?
- Am I letting others prevent me from pursuing my goals, ambitions, and desires? Do I allow my work colleagues to unfairly take advantage of me?
- Am I following my innermost feelings when making decisions, or am I afraid of the consequences? Am I making my life less enjoyable and more stressful by not following my innermost feelings?
- Am I fortifying and empowering myself?

One of the symptoms

of an approaching nervous breakdown

is the belief that one's work is terribly important.

Bertrand Russell

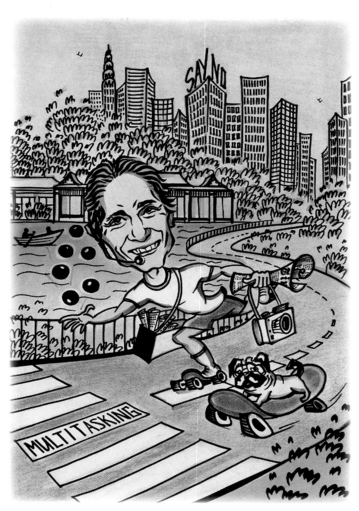

Just say No.

The power of affirmations should

never be underestimated.

They will dispel the negative and

*reinforce the positive.*PH

STEP 4

AFFIRMATIONS

THE POWER OF POSITIVE THINKING

All that we are is the result of what we have thought.
The mind is everything. What we think, we become.
Siddhartha Gautama

How is your inner dialogue
molding and shaping your life?

I have spent many years practicing meditation, but it was the practice of affirmations that I found most helpful during my period of rebuilding myself, and this is still the practice that I find most helpful today. Our minds have been programmed by a lifetime of patterns and reinforcement, and this programming has a profound effect on our choices and our attitude. I remember my amazement at witnessing the advanced nature of the ancient Greeks' understanding of healing when I was traveling and observing the ruins of the ancient Asklepieion in what had been the city of Pergamon. Patients would lie in the center of the huge domes while the Greek doctors would treat their patients simply by talking to them continuously, telling them that their health was improving and that they were growing in vitality. Inspired by this, and in the midst of my own recovery from my breakdown, I developed my own affirmation routine. Drawing on my previous experience with meditation and affirmations, this practice became, and remains, an essential element in my wellness regimen.

The affirmation process described in this step, which should be practiced daily, brings about a strong sense of calm, relaxation, and contentment. It breaks the cycle of negative thinking and supports the development of success, optimism, positivity, confidence, healing, and wellness. Practicing this technique reprograms the mind and body, allowing them to release unwanted habits and tendencies while supporting positive change. This also enables you to more effectively overcome stress. We have all been following programming of some sort for many years: what's "wrong" with us, how we "should" be, how we've made too many mistakes, or that we've failed. As we carry this negative baggage around with us in our subconscious, it seeps into all that we do, hampering our ability to make changes and move forward. Conversely, positive affirmations help us to discover contentment in the current moment and the joy of being alive right now. In essence, we are reprogramming ourselves by deleting an old negative program and replacing it with a new positive one that more accurately reflects our true nature. **Affirmations support us in more frequently discovering the power of the present moment, freeing us from our need to dwell so often in the past and future.** This is one of the most potent agents of change in your life.

The greatest weapon against stress is our ability to
choose one thought over another.
William James

〜〜〜〜

The mind is very powerful, and it needs to be spoken to. We are all aware of the power of being told, for example, that we look well; it often immediately evokes the feeling of being well. We are influenced by what people say to us. In the same way, it is extremely powerful for us to direct our bodies and minds to what we want for ourselves. We must reaffirm and say what we want for ourselves, making it known consciously and putting it out there. It is our responsibility to identify what we want and need and to ask for this from the universe. We can then both consciously and subconsciously work toward achieving that reality.

Affirmations: The Process

Although meditation is traditionally practiced in a seated position, I find lying down or *Sayana meditation* to be most beneficial, as it is the most restful position and fosters healing and rejuvenation for the mind and body. When I was exhausted with anxiety and depression, I would lie down and meditate, this being the position where the least amount of energy is expended. This position has the added benefit that it discourages any interruptions. I still practice affirmations every morning and night.

You may either sit or lie flat on your back with your eyes closed. If you happen to fall asleep, then begin focusing on your affirmations after waking. Do your best to practice in a quiet environment, free of interruptions. The early morning, before your morning walk or exercise (discussed in the following step), is an excellent time to practice affirmations. Nighttime, immediately before sleep, is also a potent time for affirmations, as it helps to reconfigure your subconscious mind as you drift off to sleep. In this way, you make your own powerful words the last thing you are aware of from the day, carrying you forward with clarity and positivity into the day that lies ahead. Think of the child being taught to pray at night, before going to sleep. Regardless of which religion or spiritual tradition is followed, this practice of gratitude for life's blessings and asking for what is desired is powerful. Harnessing the power of positive thinking just before sleep and on waking is ideal.

You may also practice affirmations during a lunch break, at work, or when you are simply taking time out or walking. It's important to find the time to say these affirmations on a daily basis. You may even do this more than once each day, if time and your desire to do so permit it. This should be a source of energizing reinforcement. It can be helpful to keep a journal of your chosen affirmations with you at all times so you can easily refer to them when you have a spare moment or want a simple reminder. Sometimes, without even reading the journal, its mere presence in your pocket can be all the reinforcement that you need.

*Conceive. Believe. Achieve.*PH

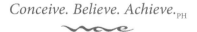

Spend some time each day focusing on your affirmations, repeating them silently. There is no need for your mouth to move or for you to make any sound, as long as you can feel the words in your own mind. However, if you would like to speak the affirmations out loud, then do so.

Choose whichever affirmations feel most resonant and relevant to you. You may create your own or draw from the suggestions below. You will also find that the particular affirmations that you are drawn to may change over time, so feel free to modify your routine as you see fit.

Suggested affirmations

With all the suggested affirmations, say the words in *italics* in your mind, feeling their meaning and power throughout your being. Feel free to modify any of the suggestions to better suit your needs.

Affirmations for the mind:

"I, [insert your name], am more powerful in this moment than I have ever been before in my life."

The power we are affirming is not a material power but your own personal power. It is about you becoming stronger as an individual, little by little, each day.

"I, [insert your name], am compassionately loving myself and forgiving myself for everything."

We all make mistakes, but we need to be kind to ourselves and not beat ourselves up over regrets. We all have life experiences that we are here to learn from, and it's only natural that we make mistakes. This is how we learn, hoping that we will not repeat the same mistakes over and over again.

"I have the strength, courage, and wisdom to make the right decisions, for myself, for the people I love, for all humankind, and for all life."

"I have the strength, courage, and wisdom to face the challenges of life, no matter what they may be; I wish to have the strength, courage, and wisdom to get up again when I fall and to never give up."

"I have the strength, courage, and wisdom to treat people the way I would like to be treated if the roles were reversed."

"I am happy, positive, and following my innermost feelings."

You might also add affirmations to support you in the changes you are working on:

"I have the strength, courage, and wisdom to talk to [insert someone's name] about [insert the particular issue]."

"I have the strength, courage, and wisdom to address the issues of [insert any particular issues you are working on]."

"I have the strength, courage, and wisdom to overcome my habit of [insert a habit or destructive coping mechanism you are freeing yourself from]."

Affirmations for the body:

This is an advanced affirmation I use, which is excellent for supporting optimal health or if you are dealing with a particular physical or psychological condition. It gives you an idea of the limitless possibilities of affirmations; you can create an affirmation for any area of life that you wish to address.

"I am grateful for my life. I'm grateful that I'm alive today at this moment. Every cell of my body is rejuvenating and in a state of perfect health. My stress, anxiety, depression [insert whatever else you would like to be free of, such as a habit or emotional pattern] is leaving my upper jaw, my lower jaw, my eyes, my nose, my sinuses, my throat... [continue listing and being aware of all of your body parts]."

During this affirmation, slowly move your awareness through every body part, focusing your attention on each area. Your gratitude may be directed to whatever you feel is appropriate, whether that's your body, life, the universe, God, yourself, or perhaps simply an expression of gratitude for being alive.

If you are experiencing any illness, address this as well. For example, when I was recovering from my breakdown, I would ask for the chemical imbalance in my brain to correct itself, saying, *"The neurochemistry in my brain is balanced and healthy. I am healthy and well."*

After first practicing these affirmations for a period of weeks during my recovery, I noticed a pronounced difference in both my body and in my outlook on life. As with each of the steps, they are a powerful agent of change and will offer great benefits if practiced daily.

With awareness and mindfulness,
*everything in life has a clear meaning.*PH

Meditation

Although affirmations are perhaps more immediately effective, meditation is also a powerful tool for well-being. Affirmations and meditation are an essential part of the Nine Natural Steps. Since my recovery, I have practiced meditation after finishing my affirmations, and I find it useful in supporting both spiritual and physiological (including neurochemical) balance.

The purpose of meditation is to experience and be aware of the silence that exists when the constant "chatter" and "noise" of the mind ceases. By becoming more acquainted with this silence you develop an awareness, where a true stillness and tranquility are revealed. [24]

The heart of spiritual practice is the cultivation of inner silence, a quietening of our thoughts, that gradually grows in our daily lives. The essential nature of our consciousness is joyful silence; this is what underlies the mind and what is experienced when our rapidly moving thoughts which are like a monkey jumping from branch to branch, becomes still. It is an infinite storehouse of peace, joy, creativity, and wellbeing.

People who have cultivated this inner silence not only experience these qualities themselves, but also radiate them to others and to their surroundings.

Meditation may have the effect of revealing to us that we are not ultimately the mind, the emotions, or the body, and that fulfilling the desires of the mind will not bring a lasting sense of contentment. All of this eventually changes the way we act in our everyday lives. Through this practice, you may begin to sense what is meant by the power of awareness,[25] the subject of Step 8. This is a powerful way to gradually free your mind from the symptoms and dangers of stress and to discover true peace and contentment. Meditation also offers numerous physical health benefits.

Breaking the cycle of negative thinking,
prevents our thoughts jumping to the past,
feeling anxious of the dreams we have of the future,
and helps each one of us stay focused
on the present and now.[PH]

Meditation: The Process

Meditation should be practiced in a quiet environment, free of distractions. Start by lying down or sitting in a comfortable position, closing your eyes, and experiencing a few gentle, natural breaths. This meditation technique uses the breath as the focal point to interrupt the constant stream of the mind. My typical process is to transition from affirmations to a place of meditation in the same session, and I highly recommend this approach.

Breathing normally through your nose, turn your attention inward, feeling the inhalation and exhalation. Keep your attention focused on your breath, and simply "watch" the breath with your awareness. Whenever a thought arises, gently return your attention to observing the breath. "Watching" the breath means to simply observe what is happening, without judgment, analysis, or reaction.

Thoughts will arise; whenever you notice that you have become lost in thought, return your attention to watching the motion of your breath. In this way, the constant stream of thoughts that is ordinarily experienced is continuously interrupted, revealing moments of silence. The more you practice, the more you will experience the peace and contentment revealed in this stillness.

If you find it difficult to focus on the breath, try using a repeated word instead. It is best that the word you choose has no inherent meaning to you but is neutral. The word "om" is often used and will be suitable if you feel comfortable with it. To employ this technique, simply replace watching the breath with repeating the word "om." Say or "hear" the word silently in your mind at a comfortable rate, and whenever you notice yourself getting distracted by thought, gently bring your attention back to slowly repeating "om" in your mind.

Continue the above technique for a predetermined amount of time. A good starting point is twenty minutes. Using a timer can be helpful to avoid needing to check the time during your meditation. The goal is to focus fully on your session, knowing that you will be notified at the completion of the time period.

Practicing Optimal Breathing

Additionally, it is highly beneficial to take some time in your day to ensure that you are breathing fully. A common response to stress is for our breathing to become shallow and driven by the accessory breathing muscles of the upper chest. Optimal breathing, however, is free from upper-chest tension and relies on the natural movement of the diaphragm, which displaces the organs of the belly to make room for the full downward, three-dimensional expansion of the lungs. To encourage this full, natural flow of breath, place one hand lightly on your upper abdomen and the other lightly on your sternum. Gently exhale, allowing the "stale air" in your lungs to leave your system. On the inhalation, allow oxygen to enter your nose and fill your lungs. The majority of the movement should be felt by your hand resting on your belly, as the diaphragm fully extends and draws the fresh air into your lungs. Exhale gently and fully, expelling the carbon dioxide from your body to make room for the fresh air on the new breath. You may integrate this into your meditation time, or simply take time out to examine your breathing and support its optimal functioning. Take a moment for yourself: natural breathing, affirmations, and meditation help to release stress and set you free.

> *By becoming masters of the direction*
> *in which our thoughts proliferate*
> *we can achieve true freedom.*
> Siddhartha Gautama

The optimist sees the rose and not its thorns;

the pessimist stares at the thorns,

oblivious to the rose.

Kahlil Gibran

SUMMARY

STEP 4 : Affirmations

- Spend time daily focusing on your affirmations, saying them to yourself and feeling them working in your mind and body.
- Use whichever affirmations feel most appealing to you, whether these are drawn from the suggestions or are created on your own.
- Practice your affirmations in a quiet place, free of distractions and interruptions, whenever possible.
- Break the cycle of negative thinking. Relearn, rethink, remold and reshape yourself.
- If you feel drawn to meditation, spend some time each day practicing the suggested technique.

Questions to ask yourself:

- What do I currently tell myself in my daily life? What patterns do I reinforce by the words that I say to myself? Are these reinforcements helping me, and if they are not, how can I reprogram them?
- What kind of outlook and what kind of experience do I want to reinforce in my life? Can I introduce this into my thinking and subconscious by including this in my daily affirmations practice?
- Am I fortifying and empowering myself?

Connect with nature.

Seize the urban gym or the great outdoors.

Breathe, feel free,

*and allow your senses to come alive.*_{PH}

nae

STEP 5

EXERCISE

Walking is man's best medicine.
Hippocrates

Are you exercising effectively enough
to break the cycle of stress?

Step 5 is a practical change that can immediately be applied on a daily basis, offering tremendous benefits in fortifying and empowering you against stress. Although it is one of the simplest steps and one that already has a place in many people's lives, it is very effective in conditioning the body and mind while also releasing stress.

I strongly recommend that you include this step with your initial practice of the nine natural steps. If you choose to begin with a single step, consider making this that step; if you choose to begin with three steps, then include this step among those three. The body is constantly being challenged on a cellular level by inflammation, immune system weakness, structural weakness, and the potential onset of degenerative diseases. Step 5 works with the nine natural steps collectively to fortify the body and mind and prevent the symptoms of stress from arising.

Consistent, sustainable exercise is essential for keeping the body in a healthy state of balance. It's important that you do something that feels natural for your particular body. If daily exercise is not already part of your routine, then ease your way into this step so as not to strain the body or deplete your energy early on. After a period of conditioning, your resilience to stress will begin to improve, and you will also notice the therapeutic effects of exercise and its role in cleansing your mind and body of stress.

Exercise is vital in combating stress. If practiced correctly, exercise has the ability to very effectively help mitigate the symptoms and dangers of stress and balance your neurochemistry.

Exercise Your Right To Walk

Daily walking was one of the most important components in my learning to master stress and in curing myself following my breakdown. Walking is the most natural form of exercise for humans; our evolutionary makeup is built for it. This is why I am a strong advocate of a brisk, uninterrupted daily walk for at least thirty to sixty minutes. Although I support and encourage any form of exercise that an individual finds enjoyable and useful, I strongly recommend embracing the following walking program for optimal health and to achieve maximum benefit from the nine steps.

As the father of modern medicine, Hippocrates, said, "Walking is man's best medicine." Although I tried many different forms of exercise while I was rebuilding myself, such as running, cycling, and swimming, after much research and trial and error, I've concluded that walking is the most effective and natural mode of exercise for the maintenance or restoration of neurochemical balance. I was first motivated to study the benefits of walking while observing my paternal grandmother's transformation after the death of her husband, when she adopted a daily walking practice. She had been overweight for as long as I could remember. I was impressed, however, by her increased vitality and the amount of weight she lost from her daily walks. She ended up maintaining excellent health right up until her death at the age of ninety-six. Having now experienced the benefits of daily walking myself, I am sure that this component of her lifestyle contributed greatly to her robust health.

The human body was clearly not built to fly or swim, as is evident when comparing our makeup to that of a bird or a fish. On closer examination, it also is apparent that we were not built to jog or run long distances, which places our joints under a high amount of strain. While the origins of running, for humans, lie in the fight-or-flight mode, running has grown in popularity as a form of exercise; more than 425,000 Americans ran a marathon in 2010, up 20 percent from the year 2000.[26] While it clearly requires dedication and the building of a strong, healthy body to run a marathon, the *New York Times* reports that 90 percent of people who train for a marathon sustain some type of injury in the process.[27] The benefits of running and any other form of exercise must be weighed against the costs, and it is up to each individual to decide what suits his or her needs. Having been a long-distance runner as well as a hurdler and sprinter at school and having had a continued interest in exercise and sport all my life, I am aware of the benefits and costs of different forms of exercise. I have thoroughly researched and tested various modes against one another.

Daily walking to promote health is going back to basics, supporting the body in the most natural and effective way. Consider other forms of exercise and how there is a limit to how long one can continue for at a time, whereas, when it comes to walking, people are able to walk comfortably for hours at a time, further evidence of walking being the optimal exercise for sustainable enjoyment and benefits. Just as Chinese healers utilize nerve endings in the feet to promote overall wellness, walking stimulates those same 7,200 nerve endings that connect to every part of the body, helping to balance your entire system, including your neurochemistry (see Appendix D, page 321). Walking is also very beneficial for diabetics and others suffering from neuropathy, a condition affecting the peripheral nervous system in which the feet and other areas can become numb or painful. Longevity studies often reveal that those living the longest tend to walk daily as a form of exercise, well into their golden years.

Walking and exercise prevent
the rusting of the mind and body.[PH]

Paul's Brisk Aerobic Walk

The simplest and most effective way to implement Step 5 is to walk briskly for at least thirty to sixty minutes every day, on your own, without interruption.

Walking is the best possible exercise.
Habituate yourself to walk very fast.
Thomas Jefferson

The walking I advocate is both anabolic and catabolic, and it activates Central Pattern Generators (CPGs) that are beneficial to our neural networks.[28] This kind of brisk, aerobic walk doesn't allow for any distractions such as talking with friends, using a cell phone, or listening to music, and it is certainly not compatible with watching TV on a treadmill. Any such activities should take place outside of your primary walking time and should not steal away from time to focus and reflect within yourself; this is *your* time. Walking with a friend or a dog may prevent you from walking at your optimal pace and should be done at a separate time as a leisure activity. Similarly, music may occupy your mind, preventing you from being with your own thoughts and giving your attention to your breathing, your exercise, and to the natural environment. This increases your lung capacity, fitness level, and supports neurochemical balance. Making a daily practice of walking is a very powerful step to take in your life. Later, once your body has been strengthened and cleansed by your walking program, you may choose to walk three to four times a week.

If possible, immerse yourself in the natural environment, whether walking on grass, on sand, in a forest, by a riverbank, or in a park. The undulating surface of the natural environment is stimulating and invigorating for the body and the central nervous system. Nature is what the body and mind have developed to expect. Your walk should always be enjoyed outside so that you can breathe the fresh air and embrace the natural environment in natural light.

If possible, try to avoid wearing sunglasses if you are walking before nine a.m. as this allows for greater stimulation of the eyes' photoreceptors and, in turn, more beneficial stimulation of the pituitary and pineal glands. This supports production of serotonin and, subsequently, melatonin, which helps to boost your mood and harmonize your sleeping patterns. The turnover of serotonin by the brain is lowest in winter[29] as the rate of production of serotonin by the brain is directly related to the prevailing duration of bright sunlight and rise rapidly with increased luminosity. The serotonin production is dependent on the duration of light exposure of the previous summer (a form of hibernation).[30] There is evidence to support that the changes in releasing serotonin by the brain underlie mood seasonality. Sunlight plays an important role in the regulation of our mood, as evidenced by the phenomenon of Seasonal Affective Disorder (SAD) that is observed in the winter months.[31]

Deeply inhaling fresh air while you walk supports the full oxygenation of your blood and, in turn, of your brain, promoting vitality, clarity of mind, and fortification against stress. This is indeed a joy to be treasured in life. Additionally, sunlight is an irreplaceable source of vitamin D, which is produced by our bodies as a response to our skin's exposure to the sun.[32] Vitamin D is essential for our health on a number of levels, including production of serotonin in the maintenance of our immune system, bone health, and the prevention of various forms of cancer.[33] The circulating vitamin D3 hormone Calcitriol, is important in the absorption of calcium from the gut to the blood, and removing calcium from the bones into the blood as it is needed for the metabolic shift. It is very important we keep walking, as it is a excellent natural weight bearing exercise, and helps keep the bones strong, and prevents osteoporosis.[34] The reality is that many of us do not live near a beach or a forest, so use a nearby park or sidewalk when needed, and enjoy your walk. Even in the concrete jungle of Manhattan, I have walked consistently through summer and winter between six a.m. and seven a.m. Heading out early avoids traffic, and despite the urban background of noise and skyscrapers, it still offers much more than a treadmill in an enclosed gym. Don't let a little rain or cold deter you from your walk; dress appropriately for the conditions, and do your best to walk outside whenever you can. Even though I miss walking barefoot on the beaches of Santa Monica, Sydney, and Auckland, I still make the most of my surroundings by heading straight for Central Park every morning, enjoying every moment of this alone-time and the serotonin boost that this natural form of exercise provides.

The ideal time to exercise is early in the morning, in part because this is when cortisol (the stress hormone) levels are highest. I encourage you to put aside this time to begin your day, which prepares you for the rest of the activity to come and allows you time for reflection. Do your best to ensure that your hour of walking is continuous, as pauses will limit the aerobic benefits and the stimulation that the exercise provides.

Your morning walk should be brisk, close to your maximum speed, with your elbows bent and hands swinging up to eye level (in a "running motion") if you are able. Bent elbows allow you to swing your arms fast without discomfort, as if you are running. (To view a video demonstration visit www. StressPandemic.com.) This gives you comprehensive physical exercise as you engage both the upper and lower body; the activity of walking in such a way works not only the muscles of the legs but the entire body, including the hips, spine, shoulders, abdomen, and arms. The head should remain level, with your eyes taking in your surroundings or focused on where you are heading but not gazing downward as if you are low on energy. The body is constantly being challenged by inflammation, immune system challenges, bone disease, and many more degenerative diseases. The nine steps, including the daily walk, help to fortify the body and mind to prevent such conditions from arising.

A sixty-seven-year-old man from Hawaii named Cyril once contacted me after reading *Stress Pandemic*. He had lost his adorable wife to cancer a few years earlier and still missed her deeply. Despite a very health-conscious lifestyle he felt lackluster, incapable of taking care of his well-being the way he used to, and he had trouble sleeping.

He seemed to eat well and was overall in good shape both mentally and physically, but a light bulb went off when I asked him about exercise. He told me he walked and watched the sunrise as he collected shells every morning on the beach. "Can you show me how you walk?" I asked him.

"What do you mean? I just walk," he replied.

That's when I got up from the table and demonstrated my walk while saying, "No, you have to really *walk*! This is a brisk, aerobic and anabolic walk that stimulates the whole body." I advised Cyril that he needed to restyle his morning walk.

Six weeks later, I received an email from Cyril telling me that he had adopted my brisk walk. The results surprised him: he was sleeping soundly and it had apparently helped elevate his spirits so much that much of his depression had lifted. He felt newly energized and felt and looked like he was in the best shape of his life. He contacted me again some time later to inform me that he had found a new life partner and that the two of them walked together each morning on the Hawaiian sand.

The difference between what most people think of as walking, and a truly aerobic, brisk walk, is significant. The walk that I advocate can have a profound impact upon your life.

> *It is remarkable how one's wits are*
> *sharpened by exercise.*
> Pliny the Younger

Stretching

I believe that any health routine should be practical and easy to embrace as a regular part of one's life. As a person with little time to waste in my own life, my exercise routine is one that can be practiced without equipment, a trainer, or a gym. Outdoor walking is consistent with this aim. So is the next important part of Step 5: stretching.

The suggested exercises can be practiced anywhere, even in a bedroom or hotel room. While living in New York, I opt for the privacy of my bedroom rather than the apartment building's gym to practice my stretches. The only equipment I require is a towel that I lay on the floor. This simplicity allows me to spend my time wisely, focused on my health and exercise rather than needing to rush from place to place and interrupting the flow of my morning.

Stretching is a natural and highly effective technique for the maintenance of the body. Just watch a cat or a dog after waking, and you will notice how it nurtures its body by stretching; nature has equipped animals to know when they should stretch. The suggested stretches will support good posture and help to avoid back pain. Stretching helps to prevent a variety of injuries throughout the body, while strengthening and conditioning your muscles, tendons, and ligaments, preventing the body from shrinking, and stimulating your overall neurochemistry. Stretching helps to release the buildup of lactic acid in the muscles, and it also helps to prevent arthritis. It aids with sleep and relaxation and promotes vitality.

The best time to stretch is immediately after your morning walk or exercise. This is another activity that you may need to ease into at first, being careful not to push your flexibility too far in the beginning.

I developed my stretching routine from yoga practices learned during my recovery from my breakdown. Although I have practiced yoga for fifteen years, I prefer to make use of this particular routine, as it incorporates the most important postures and stretches and can be practiced with ease in any environment, even a hotel room. I took the best of what I had found in traditional yoga and then refined it for simplicity and effectiveness. This set of exercises, which I practice on a daily basis for at least ten minutes, helps with restful sleep, improves your appearance, and boosts your enthusiasm for life. It also removes pain from joints and purifies the body through the use of the breath when practiced effectively, promoting harmony throughout your body.

Please visit www.StressPandemic.com to view instructions and a video for the recommended stretching routine. This set of stretches is specifically designed to give you all the benefits of practices such as yoga but in a shorter time frame and in a more convenient, practical way. For more information, please refer to Appendix A at the back of the book.

Physical fitness can neither be achieved by wishful thinking nor outright purchase.
Joseph Pilates

Earthing

Research has begun to reveal a link between health and a physical connection to the earth and its electrical field. Our bodies have developed in contact with the earth's surface. For most of our history, humans walked barefoot and slept on the ground. When footwear and clothing were first developed, it was usually of a variety that still conducted electricity, such as animal skin or hide. Scientific research is now demonstrating that this contact with the ground allows for a natural exchange of electrons between the earth and our bodies. This transfer of electrons helps to neutralize free radicals and thus can aid immensely in maintaining balance and in the prevention of disease and illness.[35]

Modern life, however, separates us from direct contact with the earth's surface. We almost always wear rubber-soled or thick-soled shoes when outdoors. We have little or no skin contact with the earth's surface in our daily lives—even children often spend little time outdoors. Children and teens spend much time with their lap tops on and mobile phones on their laps, causing increased rate of testicular cancer. Testicular cancer is the 16th most common cancer among men in the UK (2011). Children no longer climb trees or hug trees, or play with water and the garden hose and earth while doing so.

The bedding, construction, and clothing we employ completely interrupts our bodies' natural connection with the earth. This is why I recommend daily "earthing time." Earthing can be as simple as taking your morning walk barefoot, where safe and provided the environment allows it. This is often not possible, but simply standing barefoot outdoors, connected to the grass, dirt, sand, or water beneath you for five to fifteen minutes each day is enough. You could take this time to focus on your affirmations or for quiet reflection or meditation. Although not an essential part of Step 5, connecting directly with the energy of the earth, with which we have always been intimately linked, is a practice that can contribute greatly to your overall balance and well-being.

And forget not that the earth delights
to feel your bare feet and the winds
long to play with your hair.
Khalil Gibran

SUMMARY

STEP 5 : Exercise

- Exercise regularly—ideally, a brisk, aerobic walk each morning outdoors for at least thirty to sixty minutes, free of all distractions, allowing yourself time and space to reflect.
- Stretch most days (at least four), following the prescribed stretching routine or something similar.
- Ensure that you get enough exposure to natural sunlight.
- Where possible, spend fifteen minutes or more "earthing" each day, connecting directly to the earth's surface with your skin (by standing or walking barefoot).

Questions to ask yourself:

- Is my exercise routine supporting my overall health, vitality, and strength?
- Is my regular exercise a time when I can reflect on my life and the day ahead?
- Is my regular exercise simple and free of unnecessary burdens and added preparation time?
- Do I enjoy my regular exercise, and is it a part of the day that I devote to myself and give my full attention to?
- Am I practicing the 30 day LifeReStyle Process?
- Am I fortifying and empowering myself?

The doctors of the future

will no longer treat the human frame with drugs,

but rather will cure and prevent disease

with nutrition.

Thomas Edison

STEP 6

NUTRITION

Let food be thy medicine.
Hippocrates

Is my diet fortifying my body and mind?
Is it nurturing my vitality and well-being?

What we eat has a profound effect on our wellness, influencing everything from brain chemistry to sleep. Along with exercise, attending to your diet is one of the most immediately effective changes you can make in your life. A balanced and healthy diet is crucial to good health and overcoming stress. You can take a huge step forward in your overall health simply by committing to the changes outlined in this step. If you are experiencing symptoms of stress, this is one of the three most important steps to adopt initially to break the cycle of stress. As with the other steps, committing to a thirty day period of uninterrupted practice of Step 6 is the key to true transformation in this arena.

Strengthening the body and mind with optimal nutrition better equips you for dealing with stress. This also promotes a clearer, more effective mind and a more energized body, providing benefits to all areas of your life. After much research, I developed this simple and holistic approach to nutrition, giving extra attention to the effects of what we eat on our neurochemistry. Ensuring that we are supporting a healthy neurochemical balance is an important proactive step for managing stress. Our brain communicates through electrical impulses by passing neurochemicals from one cell to the next. These neurochemicals are created by the brain from the food we eat, meaning that **what we eat has a direct bearing on our state of mind. I call this effect the Good-Mood Food connection.**

I don't recommend counting calories or focusing on any one food group while neglecting others. My approach to a healthy diet is to identify health-supporting foods and eating patterns, then basing your diet around these while eliminating or greatly reducing harmful or unnatural foods and patterns. This holistic approach is far more effective and supportive of overall health than any fad or artificial measure, such as calorie counting or manipulating protein and carbohydrates. The human body is designed to thrive on a variety of natural foods. The imbalances and deficiencies in today's typical diet can only be solved by returning to the basics of nutrition by eliminating harmful and unnatural foods and ensuring that the body and mind are nourished with natural foods. Furthermore the hormone Ghrelin,[36] which is known as the hunger hormone, is secreted by the stomach and expressed in the pancreas; it is linked to appetite, weight gain and short sleep and also to impair the glucose induced insulin secretion.[37] The circulation of Ghrelin levels fall before and after a meal and stimulates appetite. When we are stressed, the Ghrelin levels rise significantly.

Research shows the circulating levels leptin is another appetite controlling hormone, it is effected by the lack of sleep. It is thought that sleep depravation plays an important role in controlling appetite. It is thought that the decrease of leptin levels, elevate ghrelin levels, as it is associated with the circadian rhythm.[38] It is known that bitter melon contains a lectin that reduces blood glucose concentrations by acting on peripheral tissues and suppressing appetite, similar to the effects of insulin in the brain. It is thought the hypoglycemic effect develops after eating bitter melon.

As with all of the Nine Natural Steps, Step 6 is supportive of and supported by all the other steps, working in conjunction to make the transition from unhealthy habits to healthy choices.

You don't have to cook fancy or complicated masterpieces—just good food from fresh ingredients.
Julia Child

Processed and unprocessed foods

Do your best to avoid processed foods and draw instead on unprocessed ingredients when preparing food. Any food that is packaged and contains a list of ingredients is processed to some degree. The more processed it is, the less natural it is, and therefore the less suitable for your body. Remember, the human body has developed over its entire history in the presence of only minimally processed foods. Our bodies, including our neurochemistry, have always thrived on these natural foods, and this is the food that our bodies have come to expect. The degree to which food today is manipulated, refined, loaded with artificial ingredients, and preserved through irradiation, pasteurization, and other technological processes has developed only within the past hundred years. Your body did not evolve to live on the typical Western diet of today; it evolved to thrive on foods that are natural and naturally prepared.

Ideally, the only processing of your food is that which you (or a healthy restaurant) do yourself immediately prior to eating, that is, combining natural ingredients and cooking them. In cases where the food you require is too inconvenient to produce from scratch yourself, such as bread, for example, choose the most natural kind available. Choose unprocessed, whole grains over refined grains, such as anything made with white flour (white bread and many other breads, white pasta, cup cakes, croissants, etc.).

Where possible, choose organic foods over conventional foods. Organic foods are produced without synthetic pesticides and fertilizers, do not contain genetically modified organisms, and are not processed using irradiation or artificial additives. All of these additives, which are often found in conventional produce and foods, can be harmful to your health in varying degrees, as they are not what the human body and brain are used to dealing with. It is best to avoid such substances as much as possible by buying organic, if and when you have the option. Additionally, unlike the modern conventional methods of recent decades, which deplete our natural resources at an unsustainable rate, organic practices are sustainable. The depletion of resources resulting from conventional farming is evident in the compromised mineral content and quality of the soil, leading to food that is less nutritious. Organic food is farmed in a natural balance with the environment, ensuring that soil quality is maintained and that the food remains as nutritious as nature intended. As an alternative to buying "certified organic" foods, it is sometimes just as effective to buy locally grown produce if you can be sure of the methods used by local farmers. Smaller producers often find the organic certification process prohibitively expensive, even if their methods are similar to those of bigger organic farmers who can afford the certification. Local food may also be fresher and more nutritious, having traveled a shorter distance than typical supermarket produce.

*Natural nutrition is your body's optimal fuel.*_{PH}

Substances to avoid:

C.R.A.P. (Caffeine, Refined Sugar, Alcohol, Processed Foods and Drinks)

Minimize or, where possible, avoid the following harmful substances:

- **Caffeine** (including coffee, tea, and high energy drinks), which artificially stimulates the body, triggering the stress response and disrupting neurochemical balance.
- **Refined sugar** (including variants such as high-fructose corn syrup), which is found in many processed foods and drinks. Also avoid artificial sweeteners.
- **Alcohol**
- **Processed foods and drinks**

To reiterate the previous section, avoid all highly processed foods, such as fast food, junk food, foods containing artificial flavors and colors, and confectionery.

It is important to avoid these substances as much as possible, as they cause harm to the body without providing any useful nutrition. For example, caffeine stimulates adrenaline (the fight-or-flight hormone), which remains in our system for a considerable length of time, throwing it out of balance. Similarly, refined sugar acts as a toxic or poisonous substance: the liver is taxed in the process of metabolizing it, potentially leading to insulin resistance, believed to be the underlying problem in obesity, type 2 diabetes, heart disease, and possibly many cancers.[39] C.R.A.P.—Caffeine, Refined Sugar, Alcohol and Processed Food and Drinks—also causes inflammation in the body and disrupts sleep patterns. Avoiding C.R.A.P. becomes all the more important when we recognize that we tend to crave sugars and fats more when we are stressed.

This is to say nothing of the numerous artificial additives that are commonly found in the processed foods addressed in the previous section. Today's processed foods may include such harmful substances as MSG, food coloring, artificial flavors, aspartame, genetically modified organisms, and nitrates, to name only a few.[40] By avoiding processed foods and instead choosing the most natural foods available, you will be doing much to avoid this toxic minefield. Learn to say No to C.R.A.P. and instead replace it with Good-Mood Foods. (Further reference Appendix B, page 294.)

Consuming C.R.A.P. will negatively impact
your neurochemistry,
and can lead to serious
*conditions of the mind and the body.*_{PH}

Meat and seafood

Keep your intake of red meat and pork to a minimum, and ensure that the red meat you do eat is lean.[41] Where possible and affordable, stick with free-range and organic meat or poultry and remove the fat content from the meat, as most toxins are stored in the fat of the animal. Instead of relying on red meat or pork, choose instead unprocessed, natural chicken or turkey, which is easier for the body to digest. Avoid organ meats (offal) such as liver, kidney, and intestine meats, as these contain high amounts of toxins. Avoid processed meats such as sausages and processed ham, which also are usually loaded with toxins, such as nitrites and environmental pollutants. Fat cells are also a storage depot for toxins in any animal,[42] thus by eating animal fat (such as that contained in beef, pork, chicken, or other animal products) you are also consuming a high concentration of toxins, which may include pesticides and hormones.

When eating seafood, choose wild-caught fish rather than farmed fish[43] where possible. Avoid seafood high in mercury—a known neurotoxin—such as tuna, marlin, swordfish, and shark. For a more detailed breakdown of seafood, refer to the food chart in the appendices.

Good-Mood Foods

are nature's magical nourishment,

opening the path to

longevity, good health, and prosperity. PH

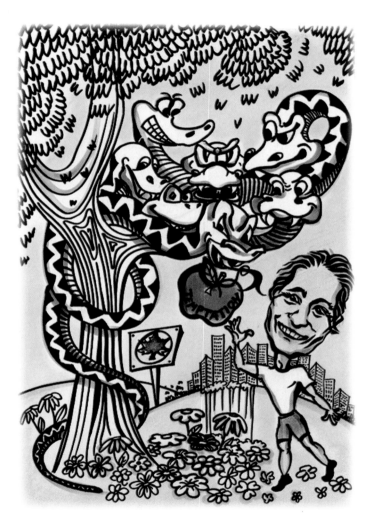

Resist temptation; things may not be
as innocent as they appear.

Dairy

Avoid dairy products, especially processed milk, cheese, cream, and butter, as much as possible.[44] Although dairy foods do contain valuable nutrients, these nutrients—such as calcium—are found in high concentrations in other foods, such as leafy green vegetables, and even freshly squeezed orange juice (see Appendix B, page 300). The negative effects of eating dairy products outweigh the benefits, due to their high animal fat content—which, as mentioned above, is a storehouse for toxins such as pesticides, fertilizers, herbicides, antibiotic residues, and veterinary medicines—and mucus-forming properties that tax the body. We need to have an awareness of diary and its byproducts, as there are trade offs of what is beneficial and what is not. We can get our calcium from other sources. There is much controversy regarding the products Type A1 or Type A2 cows.[45] It is debated that a major protein in cows – casein, causes immunological problems which lead to diabetes type 1 in humans. Many cancer treatment centers advise their patients to strictly avoid all dairy foods, and links between dairy foods and mental illness are beginning to emerge.[46] Even organically produced dairy contains naturally occurring steroids and hormones that can promote cancer growth.[47] The animal protein, fat, and cholesterol contained in dairy all contribute to heart disease, certain cancers, diabetes, and other major chronic diseases. We need to have an awareness that diary byproducts are becoming more common in the marketplace globally, and it's byproducts eg. ice cream, desserts, cheesecake, pizza etc. have addictive qualities over time. Dairy has also been found to be pro-inflammatory and, ultimately, is not a healthy choice. If you do wish to consume diary, do so in very strict moderation with awareness.

The glycemic index

Limit your intake of carbohydrates that have a high glycemic index, that is, carbohydrates that result in a relatively fast increase in blood sugar levels. These foods are quickly converted to glucose by the body and cause a spike in blood sugar levels relative to foods that have a low glycemic index. For example, replace white potatoes with brown rice or sweet potatoes. Sustained reliance on high-GI foods is linked to diseases such as type 2 diabetes and heart disease, and the sustained energy provided by low-GI foods is preferable to the burst of energy provided by high-GI foods.[48] (Refer to Appendix B, page 313 for a breakdown of common low-GI and high-GI foods.)

Good-Mood Foods to live by

Eat several servings of fresh vegetables on a daily basis, organic where possible. In addition, eat at least one serving of fresh fruit, organic where possible, daily. These are nature's healthiest and purest foods.[49] However, fruit is usually best eaten in the morning, when the body can more effectively deal with the natural sugar content, rather than in the evening or at night. Avoid bruised, overripe, or moldy fruit, as this is health-impeding for the body. If only a small section of the fruit is bruised, though, you may simply remove the contaminated portion, which is likely to contain mold.

Wash all produce before consumption, taking special care to be thorough with any nonorganic produce. It is a good idea to soak all conventional produce in a solution of water and apple cider vinegar for up to an hour (three tablespoons of apple cider vinegar to one liter of water), which helps to neutralize impurities by killing bacteria, fungi, and mold while also cleaning and disinfecting the produce. Ingesting produce that has been soaked in a vinegar solution also helps to lower the acidity of the stomach, making it more alkaline.

Eat a serving or more of raw, unsalted nuts or seeds each day, which provide essential fatty acids, protein, and other nutrients. I especially recommend almonds, walnuts, Brazil nuts, pumpkin seeds, and sunflower seeds.

Whole grains and unprocessed legumes are excellent foods for providing natural energy and strength; they are rich in protein, complex carbohydrates, and other nutrients. For further information on foods to live by (refer to Appendix B, page 294).

Eat food. Not too much. Mostly plants.
Michael Pollan

Brain Food and the Second Brain

When I was recovering from my breakdown, the doctors told me repeatedly that I had a neurochemical imbalance. Although my imbalance was serious, many of us have more minor imbalances that, nevertheless, should be addressed early rather than when it's too late. One of the components of my response to this imbalance was to research specific foods that supported production of the six main neurochemicals: serotonin, norepinephrine, dopamine, cortisol, endorphins, epinephrine and melatonin. These "brain foods" are listed in Appendix B at the back of the book.

Diet is critical to correcting and maintaining the chemical balance in the brain. The key to understanding the connection between how the food we eat affects our moods lies in our brain and body chemistry. Our brain communicates by passing chemicals called neurochemicals from one nerve cell to the next. These neurochemicals are created in the brain and body and are stimulated and formed by the food we eat. The importance of Good-Mood Foods is evident in what I call the "second brain" in the gut: 95% of our serotonin receptors are located in our gut lining, emphasizing nutrition's crucial role in our psychological well-being. By eating Good-Mood Foods and avoiding C.R.A.P., we ensure that our second brain is nourished and that our overall neurochemical balance is supported.

Water

Don't underestimate the crucial role played by water in your health. The importance of staying hydrated and providing water for the cleansing and detoxification of your system cannot be overstated. Water makes up anywhere from 57 to 78 percent of our body weight.[50] It is important in sustaining and maintaining life on an internal and external cellular level. More than anything else, water is the most important substance we consume to sustain our bodies and brains. But be careful—not all forms of liquid beverages can be counted toward our suggested daily water intake. Sodas and caffeinated teas are two sneaky culprits that can actually contribute to your dehydration rather than hydrating you. They are also toxic at a basic level due to the presence of sugar, caffeine, and artificial ingredients.

At least 75 percent of people in the United States do not drink enough water.[51] On average, a person will lose two to three liters of water per day in standard conditions and more in hot or dry weather. It is recommended that we drink two to three liters (at least eight full glasses) of water each day.[52]

Water is the elixir of life.
Atharva Veda

Drink plenty of purified, room-temperature water (chilled or iced water is less conducive to the body's natural processes), preferably water that has been purified by reverse osmosis. However, avoid drinking water with your meals, as this dilutes the digestive enzymes and impairs the efficiency of your digestive system, making it more difficult for your body to assimilate nutrients: while it is crucial to stay well hydrated, do your best to limit your intake of fluids at mealtimes to several small sips. Avoid drinking any considerable amount of water for half an hour on either side of your main meals.

The Importance of Juicing

Drinking juiced vegetables is one of the most powerful practices you can introduce to your daily routine. For one thing, the body can quickly absorb larger amounts of nutrients from juicing than from solid foods because a large part of the digestive processes necessary for whole foods is bypassed when it comes to juice. Vegetables lose nutrients and enzymes when cooked, so by juicing raw vegetables you extract a high concentration of nutrients and energy far beyond that achieved when eating cooked vegetables. Raw fruits and vegetables contain many substances that enhance health, and juicing provides the body with the most concentrated and readily absorbed source of these nutrients.

Juicing also improves the digestion and absorption of soluble fiber through the stomach and intestines and increases the breakdown of insoluble fiber by probiotic bacteria.[53] This allows you to drink the concentrated nutrition from a greater quantity of vegetables than if you were to eat the vegetables whole; therefore, you are drinking nutrition far beyond that which would be obtained through eating raw, whole vegetables. Furthermore, for most of us, our digestive system is impaired to some degree, owing to poor eating choices made over a number of years. While this limits your ability to fully assimilate the nutrients, juicing aids this nutrient absorption by "predigesting" the vegetables for you.

Raw fruits and vegetables contain many beneficial enzymes which are often eliminated by cooking processes. These enzymes play crucial roles in the body's conversion of food to energy and tissue, in metabolic processes, and in providing phytochemicals. While most people do not eat enough raw fruits and vegetables for these purposes, especially for a significant level of phytochemicals, it is relatively easy to drink enough juice to obtain sufficient amounts of these powerful nutrients. In addition, antioxidants and other immune enhancing nutrients are present in high concentrations in fresh juices. Furthermore, the concentration of antioxidants found in juices combats the damaging effects that free radicals have on skin and muscle and it also slows the onset of age-related illnesses.

Juicing nourishes your body with a flood of enzymes, vitamins, and minerals, while your cells release toxic acids in response to the alkaline nature of the vegetable juice. Waste products are then eliminated from your body through the gastrointestinal system.[54]

How to juice effectively: To juice effectively, you will need a juicer that operates at a low temperature, usually by a squeezing mechanism, to ensure that valuable enzymes are not destroyed. Juicing is best done in the morning, after your exercise. Before exercising, clean and peel your selection of fresh vegetables to ensure that you are not adding toxins to your juice. It is useful to soak the produce to be juiced in a solution of water and apple cider vinegar (three tablespoons of vinegar per liter of water), which will help to neutralize impurities and clean the vegetables, especially if some of the produce is not organic. However, because of the concentration of produce in the resulting juice, this is one area in which it is important to source organic produce as much as possible. Juice enough vegetables to produce one tall glass of juice.

After your exercise, juice the cleaned vegetables and then drink this juice fresh before your full breakfast. Fresh vegetable juice is most effective when it is consumed within twenty minutes of being extracted from the vegetables and also when consumed before, rather than after, any substantial meal. This ensures that the maximum amount of nutrients can be assimilated. I ensure that I drink my daily juice on an empty stomach by preparing and drinking it immediately after returning from my morning walk when my body is eager to absorb all the nutrition possible. I then jump into the shower and, once finished, continue with the rest of my breakfast, whether it's oatmeal, rice cereal, whole-grain rye bread, or egg whites with vegetables.

When juicing, I typically opt for a combination of carrot, spinach, broccoli, celery, red pepper, green bean, and apple for taste. You may also like to try cucumber, beet, parsley, chard, kale, asparagus, arugula, bok choy, ginger, and lemon.

Juicing is best practiced in your own home, as opposed to purchasing juice. This is because many sellers of juice use inferior ingredients that may not be fresh, organic, or properly cleaned, and they often use high-powered juicers that operate at higher temperatures and are simply not as effective as slower, higher-quality machines that better preserve nutritional value. Remember also that timing is everything—you must drink your juice within twenty minutes of extraction; thus, prepackaged or refrigerated juice is not the same. The final reason for juicing at home rather than buying juice is that the ritual itself is valuable—it requires a level of commitment, and you will find that once you make this commitment, you will be less willing to undo the health benefits of daily juicing by eating poorly at other times during the day.

Make juicing a part of your morning routine to ensure that your body receives a potent serving of fresh vegetables, that is, a potent serving of Good-Mood Foods that have absorbed energy directly from our planet's energy source: the sun's abundant radiance. This supports your system in cleansing toxins and maintaining optimal vitality, longevity and optimum health.

Tell me what you eat,
and I will tell you what you are.
Jean Anthelme Brillat-Savarin

I also recommend the following health-supporting items:

Decaffeinated green tea. I suggest drinking one cup of decaffeinated green tea (organic, if possible) after each meal to aid in digestion. Green tea aids in breaking down fats and many impurities contained in the food we eat. It also contains high amounts of the antioxidant epigallocatechin gallate (EGCG), which is believed to be a powerful fighter of many diseases. Green tea has been used to treat a number of ailments, diseases, and imbalances for thousands of years, as well as being used to assist in weight loss. I recommend drinking it daily. Coffee drinkers will find it a healthy substitute. I began drinking green tea when I was traveling to Japan for business during the 1980s, being introduced to it by author and health expert Dr. Hirotomo Ochi. Much to the amusement of my friends, these days when I travel or am out for the day, I carry tea bags with me to ensure I always have organic, decaffeinated green tea. Whether it's at a restaurant or a friend's house, it is no imposition to politely ask for a cup of hot water instead of coffee or the usual caffeinated green tea that most people stock.

Omega-3 essential fatty acids. Found in seafood and green vegetables, omega-3 fatty acids are often lacking in the typical Western diet but are essential for brain function and overall health.[55] Nuts and seeds are often regarded as good sources of omega-3 fatty acids, but they are actually better sources of omega-6 fatty acids, which are usually already in full supply in the Western diet. Two exceptions are flax seeds and walnuts which, along with seafood and green vegetables, are excellent sources of omega-3 fatty acids.

Active manuka honey is one powerful food that I recommend for its many healing properties. This is a form of monofloral honey, which is produced by bees that feed on the flowers of the manuka tree, a tea tree specific to New Zealand. It was used by the indigenous Maori people as medicine for treating fever, colds, and skin and stomach ailments. Ensure that the honey you buy is labeled "active" with a UMF value of 5 or greater.[56]

Timing your meals throughout the day

The *how* of eating is equally as important as *what* you eat. My poor eating habits developed over many years and were not dealt with until I hit a brick wall and suffered a nervous breakdown. Even though I thought I was eating good food, it was the prevalence of junk food between meals that caused real problems, not to mention the sleeping tablets, excessive amounts of vitamin supplements, and constant stress I subjected myself to. In fact, using food as a coping mechanism for stress or turning to "comfort food" can trigger allergic reactions to particular foods, while stress on its own can aggravate existing allergies.[57] In addition to this, I sometimes skipped meals or ate in unhealthily stressful situations. All this changed when I was faced with the challenge of rebuilding myself and discovered how to eat in harmony with my body's and mind's needs. On this note, I recommend the following as an example of how to eat healthily throughout the day.

Begin your day with plenty of purified, room-temperature water to aid in your body's natural cleansing and detoxification processes. I drink a liter of water before consuming any food in the morning. Drink purified, room-temperature water throughout the day, but try not to drink any significant quantity close to or during meals.

Begin preparation of your morning juice before exercising. For example, if you are juicing nonorganic vegetables, begin soaking them before beginning your morning exercise so that on completion of your exercise routine, the vegetables are ready to be juiced. Feel free to eat fruit before exercising if you feel the need for some food before exerting yourself physically.

Make and drink your juice after exercising, and then eat your full breakfast. Breakfast may consist of fruit, such as banana and berries; natural cereal or grains such as organic oatmeal (only cereals with no added sugar or artificial ingredients should be eaten), muesli, or whole-grain bread; and nuts or seeds, such as almonds, walnuts, brazil nuts, pine nuts, pumpkin seeds, sunflower seeds, flax seeds, to mention a few. If you feel the need for added protein in your breakfast, this can be achieved by incorporating egg whites into your morning meal.

For lunch, eat foods high in protein and vegetables, and incorporate complex carbohydrates such as legumes (which are also rich in protein), brown rice, quinoa, or sweet potatoes. As with all meals, try to enjoy the dining experience. Refrain from eating on the run; sit down for your meal.

Try to eat dinner close to six p.m. or seven p.m., rather than late at night. Eat some quality protein and vegetables, but try to avoid a high amount of carbohydrates; avoiding carbohydrates altogether at night can actually be very good for the rhythm of the body and its neurochemical balance. This is also the most important time to be vigilant about avoiding caffeine and minimizing or, better yet, avoiding alcohol.

Live as if you were to die tomorrow.
Learn as if you were to live forever.
Gandhi

STRESSED spelt backwards

is DESSERTS—coincidence?

I think not.

Anon.

SUMMARY

STEP 6 : Nutrition

- Eliminate C.R.A.P. from your diet, including any food containing refined sugar, artificial colors or flavors, junk food, caffeine, and alcohol.
- Avoid processed foods as much as possible.
- Minimize your intake of dairy, red meat, and pork products.
- Avoid seafood that contains high levels of mercury.
- Choose organic foods wherever possible.
- Base your diet around Good-Mood Foods, including fresh vegetables and fruits; whole grains; legumes; nuts and seeds; low-mercury seafood (wild-caught if possible); lean, unprocessed, and preferably free-range poultry.
- Drink plenty of purified, room-temperature water.
- Begin your day, after your exercise routine, with vegetable juice, made fresh and consumed within twenty minutes of juicing.
- Enjoy your meals; don't rush them.

Questions to ask yourself:

- Is my diet supporting my physical and mental health?
- Am I aware of what makes up the food I eat? Am I aware of how natural or artificial the ingredients in the food that I eat are?
- Is the food I eat natural? Am I consuming what the human body developed to thrive on? Would the ingredients that I eat have been available to humans centuries ago, or are the ingredients artificial and unnatural from my body's perspective?
- What foods can I start to eat to move towards what is natural and nutritious?
- What foods can I *stop* eating to move toward a diet that is natural, nutritious and supportive of my neurochemistry for the past 30 days?

Quality sleep heals and fortifies

the mind and body,

enabling you to successfully manage

*each challenging day.*_{PH}

STEP 7

SLEEP

*Early to bed and early to rise makes
a man healthy, wealthy, and wise.*
Benjamin Franklin

Do you wake each morning consistently feeling rested,
rejuvenated, and eager to seize the day?

The complete rest we experience during deep sleep provides
the most favorable setting for both body and mind to
truly heal and recuperate. Like many other important areas
of our health, sleep has come under pressure in the modern
world. Long working hours and disharmonious daily rhythms
disrupt the natural patterns required for a healthy mind and
body. Furthermore, stress and an unhealthy lifestyle can
jeopardize the quality and length of our sleep. An adequate
amount of sleep is needed to be able to deal with the inevitable
challenges of life and to be successful in any line of work and,
indeed, life itself.[58]

Sleep deficiency

Since the invention of the lightbulb, it has become easy for us to neglect our need for quality sleep. Many of us have allowed ourselves to get out of balance with our body's natural rhythms. Our circadian rhythms historically have revolved around sunrise and sunset, leading to an instinctive propensity to prepare for sleep with the setting of the sun. In the modern world, we are able to stay up later for whatever reason—work, socializing, various obligations—while at the same time we still must wake early in the morning for our daily commitments. This is further complicated by factors such as travel across different time zones and the resulting jet lag, which our bodies and minds are not designed to cope with; shift work, or working multiple jobs while still managing other aspects of our lives;[59] or raising infants and the associated sleepless nights, not to mention the huge burden of accumulated stress and anxiety from the day. As Part One of this book mentioned, we are in the throes of a *stress pandemic* and the modern lifestyle is taking its toll on the quality of our sleep.

Compromised sleep also disrupts the production of melatonin, a hormone secreted by the pineal gland that regulates our sleep patterns. This, in turn, alters our circadian rhythms and further prevents us from getting a good night's sleep. Ordinarily, our neurochemistry prepares us for sleep at around ten p.m., when the pineal gland's secretion of melatonin kicks in and reaches a peak at around midnight.

The natural rhythm of the hormone cortisol is for it to be secreted in the morning in relatively high levels to spur our bodies for action, and for relatively low levels to be present at night in order to allow for sleep. In an age when artificial light reigns supreme, our cortisol rhythms have shifted to a point where it's common to experience high cortisol levels at night. Our circadian rhythm—the twenty-four-hour cycle that our bodies run on—is often disrupted in our modern environment, meaning that our natural biological rhythm is confused, making quality sleep more difficult.[60]

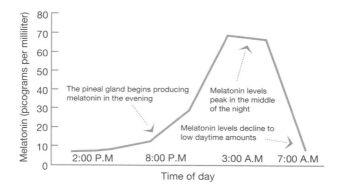

The amount of melatonin secretion from human pineal gland during various time of the day

From the graph above it can be seen that melatonin levels reach the highest value during the middle of the night and decline to the lower amounts during daytime.[61]

As a simple illustration of the role that stress and anxiety play in sleep patterns, consider how sleeping tablets—a manifestation of our inability to cope with stress levels commonly experienced today—have become one of today's most-prescribed drugs. With regard to sleeping tablets, I always like to say, "There's no pain while you're asleep"; they allow us to avoid dealing with our stress directly. Mouth guards worn while sleeping to protect against teeth-grinding, a result of stress being played out during sleep and dream time, also have become popular. Sleep difficulty is closely associated with conditions such as depression and anxiety, both of which are caused by stress, and up to 90 percent of adults with depression are found to suffer from sleep deprivation.[62] Furthermore, there is evidence to suggest that diabetes, Alzheimer's disease, and Parkinson's disease are all related to sleep deprivation. There also are people who have problems not with a deficiency of sleep but with low energy that requires them to sleep for longer than the recommended time. Regardless of which group you fall into, the Nine Natural Steps will help you restore balance and energy to your life. In this step we will deal with disruptions to quality sleep that are often encountered and show how to normalize sleep patterns. (Refer to Appendix C, page 319.)

> *Stress is when you wake up screaming, and you realize you haven't fallen asleep yet.*
>
> Anonymous

Quality sleep

It is recommended that adults sleep between seven and a half and nine hours each day.[63] The figure increases as the age of the person in question decreases, with newborns needing from twelve to eighteen hours of sleep per day.[64]

In today's fast-paced world, we often do not receive anywhere near the recommended amount of sleep. Even a minimal loss of sleep affects your energy and ability to handle stress. If you want to be at your best, sleep must be a priority; it is essential for a healthy life. The quality of your sleep affects the quality of your waking life, including your mental faculties, emotional balance, and physical vitality.

In addition to promoting overall physical and mental health and well-being, quality sleep also reduces inflammation; supports cardiovascular health; decreases the risk of cancer; improves memory, alertness, and cognitive functioning; aids in weight loss and maintaining a healthy body weight; and helps prevent depression and other mind conditions.

If you can honestly say that you experience consistently restful and restorative sleep and that your energy and alertness are satisfactory throughout the day, then you are likely receiving a sufficient amount of sleep for your needs. If you feel otherwise, or if you experience fatigue or any symptoms of stress, then it is important to make changes so that you are sleeping soundly for the recommended number of hours each night. For many years I suffered from sleep deprivation due to the demands of my work and constant travel across time zones, and this took a heavy toll. At least ninety different diagnosable sleep disorders exist;[65] sleep deprivation is a dangerous tightrope to be walking, so beware and ensure that you prioritize quality sleep.

One element that is commonly overlooked by people who have restless sleep is exercise. Daily exercise is an essential aid to quality sleep, and the brisk morning walk outlined in Step 5 is what I believe to be the most effective means of achieving beneficial exercise. At the same time, many people fail to recognize that any strenuous exercise close to bedtime can cause sleep difficulties. I have met numerous people—some who are even doctors who appear to be doing everything else right in their routines—who go running at nighttime and don't understand why they suffer from sleep difficulties. When I suggest avoiding nighttime exercise and making time for it in the morning, they usually report back to me that their sleeping difficulties have abated. Therefore, be mindful of how and when you exercise.

Keys to healthy sleep patterns

- Learn to say No to commitments that impinge upon your own personal time and space at night. There are times when urgency exists and we may need to be working or active into the late hours of the night, but this will make good sleep extremely difficult if it occurs on a regular basis. Analyze your daily routine and find the courage to say No to commitments that are preventing you from being able to relax before bed or from getting to bed at an hour that allows you enough sleep.

- Release the accumulated stress of the day before going to bed and preferably before dinner. If there are serious meetings or conversations to be had, try to schedule them in the morning or early afternoon. Do your best to cease all demanding and stressful activity by dinnertime so that you are able to enjoy a relaxing meal with minimum tension. Then, after dinner, do something that you enjoy or find relaxing. Be careful not to engage in any activity even something simple like knitting, playing cards, computer gambling, which are repetitive actions before going to bed, that may stimulate your adrenaline too much. Refrain from using e-mail or looking at a computer screen, cell phone, or tablet device, the light from which may inhibit melatonin production.

- Avoid any form of strenuous exercise late at night such as running or working out at the gym, as this will reactivate your energy and appetite, which can cause restless or interrupted sleep, such as waking at two or three a.m.

- It is also especially important to avoid eating C.R.A.P. during the evenings or at night; nighttime exercise and C.R.A.P. can interfere with the conversion of serotonin into melatonin, thus disrupting your natural biorhythms. Given that the "second brain"—containing 95% of our serotonin receptors—is located in the gut, what you eat can have a significant impact on how well you sleep.

- Honor your bedroom. The bedroom is certainly not the place for an argument, nor is it a place to watch television. Do whatever needs to be done in a different room whenever possible, ensuring that your bedroom is kept for relaxing, reflecting, loving, and sleeping.

- Ensure that your bedroom is quiet, completely dark, and at a comfortable temperature. If you find it difficult to darken your room, try using a sleeping mask or hanging darkening curtains. Daylight and its absence are detected by the pineal gland. Both sides of the day/night cycle play an important role in regulating our circadian rhythms and in the production of melatonin, thus helping us to sleep effectively.

- If you have difficulty falling asleep, try drinking chamomile tea or a short glass of hot milk with some honey (the calcium in the milk helps to relax muscles, while the honey aids serotonin and, therefore, melatonin production). Another option is to take a hot bath for twenty to thirty minutes before bed, adding Epsom salts and a few drops of lavender essential oil. Calming music, such as the sounds of tranquil natural settings, can also assist in preparing for restful sleep. If you feel restless, try using a yoga relaxation technique to calm your body and mind.

- If needed and if possible, feel free to take short naps during the day (be aware that napping for longer than half an hour may disrupt your nighttime sleep rhythm, so exercise your judgment in this). Napping has been shown to increase productivity and to support good health.[66]

- If you frequently wake during the night and find it difficult to get sustained, restful sleep, this is most likely the result of mental and emotional activity resulting from stress. Practicing the Nine Natural Steps will help you to move through these problems and balance your mind and body.

- Settle your thought processes. If you allow your brain to talk you out of committing to sleep, use the affirmations and meditation process described in Step 4.

- If you find it difficult to wake in the mornings, have something to look forward to upon waking. Yes, it might seem at first that you're forcing yourself to do something hard, but if you make it pleasurable, soon you will look forward to waking up early. Have a good reason. Set something to do early in the morning that's important such as watching the sunrise, having a hearty breakfast, meditating, or exercising.

This reason will motivate you to get up. Find something that's pleasurable for you, and look forward to it.

The close of Step 7 marks the conclusion of the Practical Steps. Before we move onto the two self-assessment steps, Steps 8 and 9, I would like to close with a story about someone very dear to my heart: my mother.

I have to begin by saying that my mother was a very challenging case. She has had a very challenging life and suffered enormous stress. She seems to have always played the role of the selfless caregiver, a person who could never say no to anyone and whose willingness to sacrifice her life to please others led me to dub her the professional care giver. I saw what this kind of stress, day in and day out, can do to someone like my mother. This is a serious issue that we must be aware of with our aging population: as we become increasingly responsible for the welfare of loved ones, we must learn to manage that responsibility.

My mother never thought that I would cure myself of my condition all those years ago, but after I did beat bipolar disorder and developed the nine natural steps, I knew I had to do what I could to help my mother. She was seventy years old, overweight, forgetful, she had been on sleeping tablets for many years, and she was forever catching colds. Her mother had suffered from Alzheimer's disease before she passed away, and I firstly encouraged my mother to walk as this would help prevent her from also developing Alzheimer's. Her response was that she already did walk her dog Hamish every day, and that she walked with friends regularly.

I bought her a plane ticket to Sydney where I was living at

the time under the pretense of inviting her to have a two week vacation with me; little did she know I was actually planning a two week boot camp! I insisted that she walk with me at six a.m. every morning. I told her to ditch the music she listened to if walking on her own and instead enjoy the sounds and peace of nature around Sydney harbor and the majestic botanical gardens. If she walked too slowly I told her I would have to chase her with a tennis racquet! She stayed with me for two weeks and immersed herself in the practical steps that I was teaching her regarding exercise, juicing, nutrition, and sleep.

Now, at age eighty-three, she is alert, capable, mobile, and very youthful for her age. She has a sharp memory and uses sleeping tablets only very rarely; she enjoys vibrant health and seldom catches colds, and is more fully in charge of her life every day as she has learned to say No in accordance with her true feelings. I'm so proud that my mother is such a shining example of nature's resilience and healing power and I hope that her example can inspire others.

*Sleep allows the body and mind
to heal and rejuvenate.*PH

SUMMARY

STEP 7 : Sleep

- Ensure that you are getting enough sleep to allow maximal recuperation and healing of body and mind. Most adults need between seven and a half and nine hours each night.
- Follow the guidelines in the "Keys to healthy sleep patterns" section in this chapter to build healthy sleep habits that will nurture your well-being.

Questions to ask yourself:

- Do I sleep restfully every night?
- Do I wake feeling rejuvenated?
- Do I get to sleep early enough each night to allow me seven and a half to nine hours of sleep?
- Am I happy with my energy levels throughout the day?
- Are any of my nighttime habits making it difficult for me to sleep restfully?
- Are there any new habits I could develop that would be conducive to more effective sleep?
- Am I fortifying and empowering myself?

Sleep is the best meditation.

The Dalai Lama

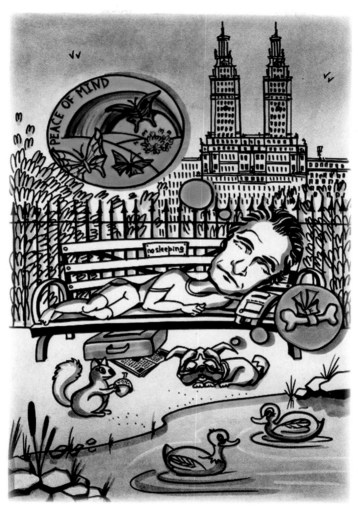

Peace of mind remains but a dream without quality sleep.

Awareness of moderation

allows you to

feel free and in control. PH

〜🖊〜

STEP 8

THE POWER OF AWARENESS

Neither can the wave that has passed by be recalled,
nor the hour which has passed return again.

Ovid

There's a line from the song "Already Gone" by The Eagles that often comes to mind when I talk about awareness: "So often times it happens that we live our lives in chains / And we never even know we have the key." Awareness is that key that will unlock those chains and set us free.

The first seven steps are powerful tools for change that will bring you into balance with your natural well-being, fortifying and empowering you against stress. By introducing these steps into your life and using them as your guide, you will see real changes in your ability to deal with inevitable challenges, both big and small, as well as in the strength and vitality of your body and mind. This progress enables you to break the cycle of stress and live fully.

The progress you make rests upon one factor more than any other: awareness. MWellA—Mind Wellness Awareness—is a name that came to me one beautiful day on Avalon Beach in Sydney, Australia. To me, it encapsulates the understanding that you can be conscious of where your mind is and the thoughts you are having and that this is the most essential link to true wellness. One can develop a strong sense of awareness and use this as the barometer for thoughts, feelings, emotions, and moods. As you develop your awareness of your thoughts and desires, of your lifestyle, and of the present moment, you will bring your body and mind back into a state of harmony with greater frequency and ease. You will cease to crave, need, and want what you don't really require as your baseline state becomes one of increasing balance and contentment.

I see the power of our awareness as stemming from two distinct areas. First, by applying your power of awareness to your thought patterns, desires, and their consequences, you empower yourself to make decisions based on wisdom. Second, as you continue your practice of the steps, your awareness of the present moment will develop and strengthen, opening the way to true peace, fulfillment, and contentment.

Awareness of your thoughts and desires

The awareness I am speaking of arises the moment you become conscious of your senses at birth and comes into play with every thought, from the very first thought you have in the morning to your last each night before sleep takes over. By engaging your awareness, you can become more mindful of your thoughts, desires, and actions, which is the ultimate key to mastering stress and is of enormous benefit in your everyday life.

The ancestor of every action is a thought.
Ralph Waldo Emerson

The moment you have a thought, a feeling is triggered. Depending on the intensity of this thought, the feeling could be lingering or brief and will also generate an emotion or a mood. Your desire is heightened by this process, and this is where we have the opportunity to employ our willpower. You have the opportunity to say No to disruptive or destructive thoughts and Yes to those that are desirable. This discernment rests upon your ability to follow your innermost feelings. As the picture of the rainbow at the end of this chapter illustrates, you must have an awareness of where your thoughts are taking you. Your awareness of your thoughts, and the strength of your willpower, play an essential role in your desires and the outcome of those thoughts. These factors determine to what degree your thoughts become feelings, emotions, moods, and ultimately actions and consequences.

In progressing toward a place of contentment, I would find it helpful to observe the links between my senses, thoughts, feelings, emotions, moods, and desires. When I was at the Menninger Clinic, I noticed how the visual stimulus of seeing other patients and sensing their depressed state gave rise to the thought that I didn't want to remain in a similar state forever. A feeling of sadness was the result of this thought. My brain's physical response was the expression of the emotion of sadness as tears streamed down my face. My mood was instantly lowered; as my serotonin levels dropped, I eventually couldn't get out of bed. My desire to free myself from the confines of the Menninger Clinic and these mind conditions grew stronger and stronger; I didn't like my surroundings and I wanted to get home to my children. I clung to this very strong desire and I had to exercise considerable willpower, which developed over time, to fulfill it. It was important for me to be aware of what had initially triggered this desire, and with this awareness of the true nature of my desire and where it would lead me, I was able to exercise my willpower and achieve my goal of returning home to my family. The awareness of the original thought was the driving force for achieving my goal.

Perhaps the most important component of this process is the ability to recognize and welcome useful thoughts and to prevent other thoughts from hijacking them. Conversely, there is great power in deciding to kill off harmful thoughts early on, before they gather too much momentum. This all rests upon the power of your awareness.

*Every action has a reaction and consequences.*_{PH}

During my recovery, I found it helpful to keep a small diary of my progress, which was a great aid for learning to monitor my state and ultimately to master my stress. It is useful to write down, on a day-to-day basis, the root causes or primary triggers of your destructive and constructive thoughts, and I suggest you incorporate this into your routine. Use this information to develop your awareness of where your desires and temptations arise from and when you should say No to these desires. It could relate specifically to one of the steps, such as nutrition or exercise, or to an aspect more specific to your particular situation. This has the effect of further supporting awareness of your lifestyle. As this awareness of your lifestyle choices grows, you will find it easier to know which choices are of benefit to you, and which are harmful.

> *Developing a sense of awareness equips you with the tools to fight back.*_{PH}

It is important to understand that most of our desires take us toward either the "dark side" or the "bright side" of life. We must use our power of awareness to monitor where our thoughts and desires are leading us—toward a place of contentment, or further away from achieving true peace of mind. Most people live in a grey area, never truly aware of the direction they are choosing. Through maintaining an awareness of your desires, your innermost feelings will help guide you in a direction where your ambition, goals, needs, and desires all come into a state of balance and allow you to find contentment. The key to taking back the power of our awareness is to be aware and mindful of the decisions we are making today.[67]

Be mindful that temptation toward the dark side will come from all directions. For example, as you refine your diet, people will still be making you your favorite dish or asking you to join them for food that is no longer of benefit to you. It is common for the people in our lives to feel threatened by our desire for change and improvement, and you may encounter resistance from them to your attempts to change as they try to keep you a party to destructive behavior and habits. It is up to you to say No to the desires that no longer lead you to the bright side of life—to contentment and peace of mind. Awareness of the equilibrium between your ambition and contentment is also essential in the management of stress; without this balance, ambition can be a harmful source of stress and poor lifestyle decisions.

*There is a point where your true ambitions, goals, and desires merge with contentment.*PH

We are constantly told through the media and through our culture what we should want, what we should have, and what we should be. You, and only you, have the power to be aware of your own innermost feelings and the nature of your desires. Awareness and mindfulness of your thoughts and desires will give you a much greater command of your life's true needs. It opens the way for you to become the true "new you" as you develop your awareness of who you really are and become the person you are meant to be. Naturally, this takes time.

It is common for much discontentment to have evolved over time due to your accumulated life experiences, molding your character and making you into the person you are in the process. The habits that have been formed are learned behavior and ultimately result in difficulty in saying No or Yes to your innermost feelings. As you develop your mindfulness and awareness, you will discover joy, harmony, and contentment. You will be able to live well. No longer a passive passenger, you will find yourself 100 percent in control and in the driver's seat in the exciting, ever-challenging journey of your life.

You should also be aware that, due to the stressors of life, our senses can become overcharged and, over time, desensitized. When you are under stress, you need to have extra vigilance and awareness. This is the time when we are most vulnerable to making unwise decisions. We are constantly adapting, but at what cost? Also of paramount importance is having an awareness that your senses may be desensitized due to emotional trauma or some unpleasant experience from the past, which may impact on the decisions that you are making at this present moment. Your "sixth sense" and your awareness coupled with mindfulness should be your barometer as to where you are at any given time.

*Be aware. Don't become desensitized.*_{PH}

Present-Moment Awareness

The natural result of progress with the first seven steps is the gradual refocusing of your awareness into the present moment. Practicing these seven steps helps you to master life and come to a state of balance, wherein you are at peace with yourself and content with life from moment to moment. Your neurochemistry becomes balanced as the cycle of stress is broken and the over-activation of the stress response is alleviated. The issues that previously lingered and dragged you back into the past eventually evaporate. Similarly, anxieties you once experienced about the future and your longing for the hoped-for happiness that you associated with obtaining certain goals don't seem to hold the overriding importance that they once did. Whereas you once hoped to find happiness by attaining certain things in the future, you come to realize that even when you achieve significant goals in your life, you have still experienced dissatisfaction and a need to reach for more very soon afterward. As you become accustomed to living in the present, your sense of contentment here and now becomes more real than your mental and emotional struggles as you begin to develop a true love for yourself and for life.

Consider the case of someone who once enjoyed very good health and then happened to develop a serious, prolonged illness. Over time, the experience of pain and discomfort becomes normal—so much so that, after years of dealing with constant illness, the person has completely lost touch with the experience of wellness and health. The body and mind tire and grow accustomed to pain over a long period of time, and they no longer know what it is like to be free of pain. This applies to all of us. It could be that, at some stage of our lives, we knew what it was like to feel free, to live in the moment, and to enjoy our lives, free of the burden of stress. We wouldn't get obsessed with the past or the future, and we were able to live in relative contentment—like a child who is perfectly loved and content, not angry at the past, and with no idea of the future, but just content to enjoy the moment. For most of us, this changes over time, with growing responsibilities and the realities of living in a competitive world. The expectations that others have for us and our desire to fit in and be accepted lead us down paths that are not in line with our innermost feelings. As time goes by, our lives become focused on ambitions and goals, causing us to forget the ease of living in a place of contentment and happiness. As we gather more life experiences and learn life's lessons, some of which can be very harsh, they have a lasting impact on us emotionally and physically.

Dwelling on our memories drags us into the past. Some of our memories could be pleasant, but most will be unresolved issues where unreleased pain is still harbored to some degree, resulting in the experience of regret, sadness, fear, guilt, and anger. Similarly, the future has a way of pulling us out of the present moment and often triggers anxiety due to the uncertainty of life and the pressure of our commitments. If given the opportunity, the mind will play out every thought and emotion continuously, preventing us from experiencing the present moment, where the biggest prizes of all are to be found: peace of mind, joy, and contentment.

Remember that each moment is transient. Whatever is happening in your life will pass. If it is bad, it will pass. If it is good, it will pass. Think of a cork bobbing on the surface of the water—it does not move or shift its position; the water below it moves. Similarly, aspire to keep your attention on the present moment while the situations and experiences of life move around you without disturbing your balance.

Practical Awareness

The nine steps are your armor and tools for dealing with the stress pandemic that is becoming so apparent around the world. Each one of us is a powerful warrior in the coliseum of life, and these steps equip us well for our challenges. The nine steps can also serve as useful points of focus for your awareness. For example, make it a practice to be aware of your decisions and whether or not you are acting from your true, innermost feelings, applying Step 3 (Learn to Say No). When engaged in any activity that begins to feel habitual, bring your awareness back to your physical and psychological health, remembering the harmful allure of destructive coping mechanisms and your desire to be free of stress and the crutches you have used to deal with it in the past (Step 2, Kick Your Bad Habits). Maintain awareness of your dietary decisions whenever engaged in eating, ensuring that you are serving your best interests and not your cravings or habits (Step 6, Nutrition). By living in this way, your self-awareness grows, and your attention becomes increasingly focused on what is most important to you in the present moment.

Building awareness in this sense enables you to develop a more accurate barometer of your well-being. Your symptoms of stress are your barometer of wellness, and as you grow in awareness, you will become more proficient in noticing these symptoms. You will find that the psychological and physical symptoms that you once had begin to lessen in intensity, and this ongoing progress becomes the barometer for your well-being. Similarly, if you notice new symptoms of stress appearing, this will also be valuable feedback that you can use to steer yourself in the direction of greater well-being. In this way, awareness will help prevent you from reaching the tipping point where stress takes you to a place of developing serious mind conditions. (Ref. LifeReStyle Stress Pyramid, page 24)

Maintain your consciousness of the present moment. Be aware that, as soon as you awake each morning, your mind will want to latch onto some thought, and it is up to you to be mindful of the consequences of your thoughts. Every thought has the potential to affect your physical and mental well-being,[68] your state, your actions, and their repercussions. Be aware of the nature of your desire, and understand the consequences and actions that spring from your desire. To be free of cravings, clinging, and desire is to experience contentment and balanced neurochemistry; evaluate your level of contentment at any given time.

The nine steps will support you in freeing yourself from the accumulated habits and injuries that have dragged you out of alignment with natural contentment. Living in the present with awareness is the ultimate result of freeing yourself from stress; however, it cannot be forced. Living in the present arises naturally as you develop a healthy way of life and deal with psychological habits that keep you in a place of stress. In time, your whole attitude toward many aspects of life will change for the better, and you won't be dependent on sorting issues out from your past or looking toward something in the future to bring you happiness and contentment. You can encourage development of this state of mind toward life by noticing where your thoughts and emotions are centered at any given time. See if you are able to bring your awareness back to this very moment and fully experience life here and now. Eventually, you will be able to love yourself fully, which comes from the willingness to fully forgive yourself and embrace the present moment.

The untrained mind is stupid! Sense impressions

come and trick it into happiness, suffering, gladness

and sorrow, but the mind's true nature is none of

those things… really this mind of ours is already

unmoving and peaceful.

Ajahn Chah

SUMMARY

STEP 8 : The Power of Awareness

- Practice the first seven steps and commit to them fully.
- Be mindful of your thoughts, your desires, and their likely consequences. Have an awareness of your lifestyle.
- Put your growing awareness of your innermost feelings, your thoughts, and your desires to good use by saying No to thoughts that don't serve you and Yes to thoughts that are of benefit to you.
- As you discover more ease and health in your life, allow yourself to embrace the present moment, enjoying fully what life has to offer, here and now.
- Notice when your awareness is unnecessarily on the past or the future, and gently bring it back to this very moment.
- Become aware of what you are holding on to, and see if you can begin to forgive yourself—to love yourself.

Questions to ask yourself:

- Where are my thoughts leading me?
- Are my thoughts leading me in the direction of the dark side of life (further from contentment and true wellness) or toward the bright side of life (closer to contentment and true wellness)?
- Where is my awareness? Is it on the past, the future, or the present?
- Can I let go of the past and the future and experience contentment right here and now?

Awareness is observation without

choice, condemnation, or justification.

Jiddu Krishnamurthi

THE LifeReStyle THOUGHT PROCESS

AWARENESS

Brain Response					
Thought					
Thought Proliferation					
Feelings		Feeling Good	Feeling Bad		
Emotions		Laughing	Crying		
Desire	Dopamine Hijack				
Moods		Good Mood	Bad Mood		
Willpower	LifeReStyle Process				
Reaction and Consquences		Awareness Peace of Mind	No Peace of Mind		

Stimulus

Hear
Taste
Smell
Sixth Sense (Instinct)
Touch
See

THOUGHT

Every proliferating thought has a result,
Every action has a reaction and consequences

"Mind jumps like a monkey from tree to tree..."

We are what we think.

All that we are arises with our thoughts.

With our thoughts we make the world.

Siddhartha Gautama

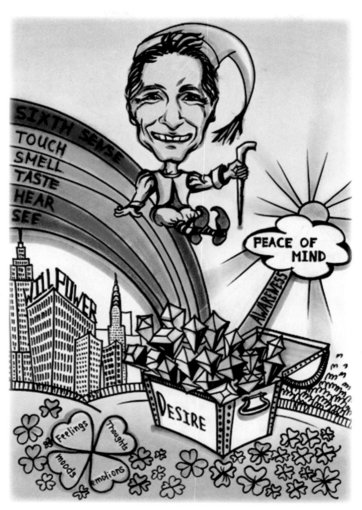

Awareness leads to mindfulness and contentment.

Never

Never

Never

Give Up.

Winston Churchill

STEP 9

DON'T GIVE UP

*Most of the important things in the world have been
accomplished by people who have kept on trying
when there seemed to be no hope at all.*

Dale Carnegie

～⌒～

No matter where you are, no matter what your situation may be, no matter what challenges you are facing, never allow your flame of hope to be extinguished. Don't ever give up. As long as you have a desire to live fully and to be free of stress, you have all the power you need. You now also have the tools. The Nine Natural Steps enabled me to break free of the accumulated stress that led to my mental breakdown and the resulting stress of living with a severe mind condition. They enabled me to live with contentment, joy, and love for life.

Hope and Commitment

The final step is one that, like Step 8, invites us into self-reflection time and again, as it directly relates to all of the other steps and to every facet of life. When we resolve to never give up, hope and commitment become the fuel that takes us where we need to go.

Regardless of where you are on the spectrum—from wishing to leave behind everyday stress, to wanting to recover from a serious mind condition—you have the power to move forward in your life. You can fortify yourself against stress and empower yourself to move to a new level in your life, one of awareness and contentment.

For the growing number of us who are dealing with stress but are not affected by severe stress-related conditions, this represents the commitment to transforming and restyling your life. A life free of harmful stress and filled with joy is your birthright, and it is this very realization, combined with your persistence, that fuels your progress and success.

For those who are dealing with severe stress-related conditions, the notions of hope and commitment include the knowledge that freedom from your condition and stigma, and the ability to live fully and with wellness, are within reach. There were many times during my recovery from my breakdown when I found it almost impossible to believe that I would ever be myself again, that I would ever be happy again. The doctors told me I would never be the same, that I would be dependent on medication for the rest of my life and that I would eventually relapse. To me, this was like being handed a death sentence. No one around me had answers to what had happened to me or what my future would hold in terms of my mental, emotional, and physical well-being. Everything that I did hear was negative. I felt ashamed; I felt a failure to myself and my loved ones; I felt alone.

Through all the ups and downs, I refused to let go of the

final ounce of hope within me. Despite the discouragement, doubt, and fear, I held onto the flame of hope deep within me—the hope that knew there was a chance, that knew it was possible for me to recover and live the life I wanted to live. I was determined to survive. I was determined to thrive. If I had given up, I never would have beaten stress and freed myself from my condition. Although there were times when all seemed hopeless, I continued with my journey and held onto whatever hope I could find.

Remember, change takes time. Breaking habits and forming new ones is not easy, and we all stumble as we begin the process of change. Take on only as much as you can handle, and don't get discouraged if you experience setbacks. You may want to choose only two steps to focus on in the beginning—such as Exercise and Nutrition—and as you become adept at integrating these steps into your life, you can move on to a third and fourth. Continue to challenge yourself as your sense of well-being and health improve and your love of life and present-moment awareness develop. You will eventually sense that you are beginning to truly establish a new way of life. You will feel it.

Never allow your flame of hope
*to be extinguished.*_{PH}

Gradually build your practice of the steps until you are implementing all steps for a sustained period of time (thirty days or more) without interruption. You can then tailor the program, especially the four practical steps (Steps 4 through 7), to meet your own personal needs. For example, once you have mastered the practical steps, you may find that you only need to do the full stretching routine every other day. Once you've achieved an uninterrupted thirty-day period of practicing the four practical steps, use your own judgment in determining what suits your needs. In time, your habits and lifestyle will change, and you will notice a profound improvement in your well-being. You will become more upbeat and optimistic as you move forward and embark on your life's great journey.

We need a sense of hope that we can learn to master stress in our lives and overcome any stress-related conditions. We must push ourselves to take the first steps. Like a child learning to walk, each of us must continue on our journey despite falling over many times, in the knowledge that we are moving in the right direction and that one day we will walk with ease. It is important that we commit to nurturing our well-being and loving ourselves enough to make our own welfare and health the priority of our lives. We can then enjoy what life truly has to offer. In doing so, we will have something of real value to share with our loved ones and the world at large.

The phoenix hope, can wing her way through the desert skies, and still defying fortune's spite; revive from ashes and rise.
Miguel de Cervantes

We all fall down, and we all face challenges every day. That is life. The courage is in trying. You are not alone. Nurture your flame of hope; don't give up.

SUMMARY

STEP 9 : Don't Give Up

- Remember that you have the power to move forward in your life, to fortify and empower yourself.
- Allow yourself time to break habits and form new ones.
- Understand that it is natural to stumble; the courage is in getting back up.
- Continue to pursue your application of the nine steps until you reach a thirty-day period of uninterrupted practice of the steps.
- Nurture your flame of hope and maintain your commitment, regardless of the challenges you encounter.

You are not alone.

You are worth it.

Have hope, it is everything,

NEVER EVER GIVE UP!

Paul Huljich

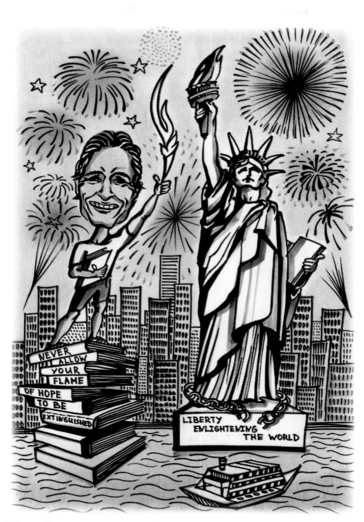

Through commitment and persistence, find your true freedom.

THE LifeReStyle DEVELOPMENT & SOLVING OF STRESS

The Stress Response: is the trigger action when we feel threatened or challenged, and causes a psychological and physiological change known as the Fight or Flight reaction; If activated constantly will cause an imbalance of the mind and the body.

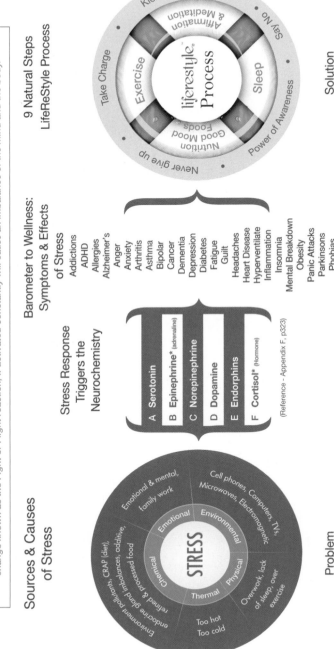

9 Natural Steps
LifeReStyle Process

Kick your bad habits

Affirmation & Meditation

Take Charge

Say No

Exercise

lifereStyle™ Process

Sleep

Nutrition Good Mood Foods

Never give up

Power of Awareness

Solution

- Cortisol x10 with exercise, x50 with STRESS
- Cortisol highest in the morning, lowest in the evening

Barometer to Wellness:
Symptoms & Effects of Stress

Addictions
ADHD
Allergies
Alzheimer's
Anger
Anxiety
Arthritis
Asthma
Bipolar
Cancer
Dementia
Depression
Diabetes
Fatigue
Guilt
Headaches
Heart Disease
Hyperventilate
Inflammation
Insomnia
Mental Breakdown
Obesity
Panic Attacks
Parkinsons
Phobias
Psoriasis
PTSD
Stroke
Teeth-Grinding
Weight issues
Worry

Stress Response Triggers the Neurochemistry

A Serotonin
B Epinephrine* (adrenaline)
C Norepinephrine
D Dopamine
E Endorphins
F Cortisol* (Hormone)

(Reference - Appendix F, p323)

Sources & Causes of Stress

Emotional & mental, family work

Cell phones, Computers, TVs, Microwaves, Electromagnetic

Emotional

Environmental

STRESS

Chemical

Physical

Thermal

Environment pollutants, CRAP (diet), refined & processed food endocrine gland imbalances, additive,

Overwork, lack of sleep, over exercise

Too hot Too cold

Problem

Kinds of stress: Chronic stress - Acute stress
Play stress (Eustress)

IN A NUTSHELL:
A NINE NATURAL STEPS CHECKLIST

Refer to these questions periodically to check your understanding and practice of the Nine Natural Steps.

- Are my symptoms of stress diminishing?
- Am I eating more Good-Mood Foods as opposed to C.R.A.P?
- Am I juicing at the optimal time for maximum results?
- Am I feeding my 'second brain' with optimal nutrition? Do I feel upbeat?
- Given that cortisol levels are highest in the morning and lowest in the evening, am I doing the heavy lifting in the morning rather than the evening?
- Are the crutches and bad habits that I lean on diminishing?
- Is my Dopamine being hijacked?
- Am I exercising at the right time and the optimal way, in the morning and not in the evening? Am I taking a brisk aerobic walk in the fresh air and stimulating the 7200 nerve endings in my feet?
- Am I getting enough Vitamin D from sunlight?
- Am I practicing my positive affirmations to fortify and empower myself and to cope with this day?
- Am I sleeping well?
- Am I feeling bullied, am I learning to say "No"?
- Am I following my true innermost feelings?
- Am I in charge of my life? What am I not in charge of? What am I doing about it?
- Is my stress response being over-stimulated?
- Am I implementing the thirty-day LifeReStyle process without a break?

Watch your thoughts; they become words.

Watch your words; they become actions.

Watch your actions; they become habits.

Watch your habits; they become character.

Watch your character; for it becomes your destiny.

Lao Tzu

SUMMARY OF
THE NINE NATURAL STEPS

This section is provided not only to summarize what you have just read but also for your future reference. It is intended as a quick-reference guide for you to refresh your understanding of any or all of the steps' main points.

THE TRANSFORMATIVE STEPS

Steps 1, 2, and 3 are the transformative steps, designed to address the underlying habits that are the cause of stress. While these steps are essential, they are also steps that you will master gradually and continuously. They are not activities that you can engage in and then move on with the rest of your day; they are tools that enable you to shift your attitudes and overcome the causes of stress, and as such require continual practice, exploration, and development. You will get better and better at using these tools the more you apply them. These first three steps are the keys to true personal transformation.

STEP 1 : Take Charge

- Know that you deserve well-being and balance.
- Accept the need for change—recognize that the "old you" has caused stress.
- Take charge—take responsibility for making changes and implementing the nine steps of the LifeReStyle Process.
- Be aware of any symptoms of stress arising in your life.
- Make time each day for putting the nine steps into practice.
- Renew your commitment every time you fall. Take charge and stay in charge.

Questions to ask yourself:

- How do I create stress in my life?
- How do I respond to challenges and stressful situations?
- How do I maintain my body and mind to be able to withstand stress?
- Am I aware of where I am in my life right now?
- Am I aware of any symptoms of stress in my body and mind?
- How do I use my time? Am I using my time efficiently so I can put these changes into action?
- Am I fortifying and empowering myself?

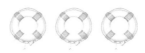

STEP 2 : Kick Your Bad Habits

- Observe how you spend your time, noticing if certain patterns feel more "addictive," or like a "release," than enjoyable.
- Consider whether or not these patterns are harmful to your well-being or limit your true enjoyment of life.
- Resolve to overcome your destructive coping mechanisms, beginning with one at a time and taking on what you can comfortably manage as you free yourself from harmful habits. Free yourself from the dopamine hijack of addictive patterns and destructive coping mechanisms.
- Gradually decrease your dependence on each addictive pattern, monitoring your daily progress in writing.
- Continue monitoring the addiction until you have completed a thirty-day period of total independence from the pattern.
- Recognize that beating addictions takes time and can be challenging and that your practice of all of the nine steps will assist in freeing you from destructive coping mechanisms.

Questions to ask yourself:

- How reliant am I on my habits?
- Are there patterns I turn to when I'm stressed?
- If so, are these activities a crutch, and am I using them to avoid or mask stress?
- Am I enjoying things in moderation, or am I being excessive?
- How do these habits affect my life and well-being?
- Am I fortifying and empowering myself?
- Am I breaking my bad habits following the 30 day LifeReStyle process?

STEP 3 : Learn to Say No

- Learn to say No to demands and requests that are not in line with your true desires. Don't commit to obligations that you do not have the necessary time and energy for.
- Learn to discern your innermost feelings.
- Record decisions that you've made and how you made them so you can learn from their outcomes at a later date and compare similar situations in the future.
- Practice following your innermost feelings so that regardless of whether things work out the way you want them to, you know that you have done your best and been true to yourself.

Questions to ask yourself:

- Am I agreeing to something, taking on a commitment, or prioritizing someone else's wishes, while not truly wanting to?
- Do I have the necessary time and energy to devote to commitments that I don't feel strongly about, or are they causing substantial and unnecessary stress in my life?
- Am I letting others prevent me from pursuing my goals, ambitions, and desires?
- Do I allow my work colleagues to unfairly take advantage of me?
- Am I following my innermost feelings when making decisions, or am I afraid of the consequences? Am I making my life less enjoyable and more stressful by not following my innermost feelings?
- Am I fortifying and empowering myself?

THE PRACTICAL STEPS

Steps 4, 5, 6, and 7 are the practical steps. The function of these steps is to optimize your general wellness and allow you to feel better than you've ever felt before. By strengthening body and mind, they enable you to deal more effectively with stress, assist in the release of stress both physiologically and psychologically, and help maintain a healthy neurochemical balance. These steps can be integrated into your daily routine and then tailored to your particular needs. For example, during periods of greater pressure and stress, you may find yourself needing to be extra vigilant about daily stretching and avoiding all toxic foods. However, if you have built the practical steps into your daily routine and after some time find yourself not needing to stretch every day, for instance, feel free to stretch only three or four times a week during less challenging times. Use your judgment in assessing what is best for you, after you have already succeeded in implementing the practical steps into your daily routine.

*Say No to stress and live stress free.*_{PH}

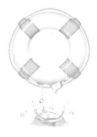

STEP 4 : Affirmations

- Spend time daily focusing on your affirmations, saying them to yourself and feeling them working in your mind and body.
- Use whichever affirmations feel most appealing to you, whether these are drawn from the suggestions or are created on your own.
- Practice your affirmations in a quiet place, free of distractions and interruptions, whenever possible.
- Break the cycle of negative thinking. Relearn, rethink, remold and reshape yourself.
- If you feel drawn to meditation, spend some time each day practicing the suggested technique.

Questions to ask yourself:

- What do I currently tell myself in my daily life?
- What patterns do I reinforce by the words that I say to myself?
- Are these reinforcements helping me, and if they are not, how can I reprogram them?
- What kind of outlook, and what kind of experience, do I want to reinforce in my life?
- Can I introduce this into my thinking and subconscious by including this in my daily affirmations practice?
- Am I fortifying and empowering myself?

STEP 5 : Exercise

- Exercise regularly—ideally, a brisk, aerobic walk each morning outdoors for at least thirty to sixty minutes, free of all distractions, allowing yourself time and space to reflect.
- Stretch most days (at least four), following the prescribed stretching routine or something similar.
- Ensure that you get enough exposure to natural sunlight.
- Where possible, spend ten minutes or more "earthing" each day, connecting directly to the earth's surface with your skin (by standing or walking barefoot).

Questions to ask yourself:

- Is my exercise routine supporting my body's overall health, vitality, and strength?
- Is my regular exercise a time when I can reflect on my life and the day ahead?
- Is my regular exercise simple and free of unnecessary burdens and added preparation time?
- Do I enjoy my regular exercise, and is it a part of the day that I devote to myself and give my full attention to?
- Am I fortifying and empowering myself?

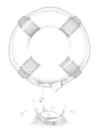

STEP 6 : Nutrition

- Eliminate C.R.A.P. from your diet, including any food containing refined sugar, artificial colors or flavors, junk food, caffeine, and alcohol.
- Avoid processed foods as much as possible.
- Minimize your intake of dairy, red meat, and pork products.
- Avoid seafood that contains high levels of mercury.
- Choose organic foods wherever possible.
- Base your diet around Good-Mood Foods, including fresh vegetables and fruits; whole grains; legumes; nuts and seeds; low-mercury seafood (wild-caught if possible); lean, unprocessed, and preferably free-range poultry.
- Drink plenty of purified, room-temperature water.
- Begin your day, after your exercise routine, with vegetable juice, made fresh and consumed within twenty minutes of juicing.
- Enjoy your meals; don't rush them.

Questions to ask yourself:

- Is my diet supporting my physical and mental health?
- Am I aware of what makes up the food I eat? Am I aware of how natural or artificial the ingredients in the food that I eat are?
- Is the food I eat natural? Am I consuming what the human body developed to thrive on? Would the ingredients that I eat have been available to humans centuries ago, or are the ingredients artificial and unnatural from my body's perspective?
- What foods can I *stop* eating to move toward a diet that is natural and nutritious?
- What foods can I *start* eating to move toward a diet that is natural and nutritious?

STEP 7 : Sleep

- Ensure that you are getting enough sleep to allow maximal recuperation and healing of body and mind. Most adults need between seven and a half and nine hours each night.
- Follow the guidelines in the "Keys to healthy sleep patterns" section in this chapter to build healthy sleep habits that will nurture your well-being.

Questions to ask yourself:

- Do I sleep restfully every night?
- Do I wake feeling rejuvenated?
- Do I get to sleep early enough each night to allow me seven and a half to nine hours of sleep?
- Am I happy with my energy levels throughout the day?
- Are any of my nighttime habits making it difficult for me to sleep restfully?
- Are there any new habits I could develop that would be conducive to more effective sleep?
- Am I fortifying and empowering myself?

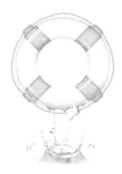

Living the Practical Steps in a Typical Day

The following is provided as an example of how the four practical steps might be applied on a daily basis.

■ On waking

While lying in bed, or after rising, spend some time on affirmations or meditation.

Begin your day with plenty of purified, room-temperature water to aid in your body's natural cleansing and detoxification processes.

■ Morning

Begin preparation of your morning juice by soaking produce so that it's ready for juicing after your exercise routine. Feel free to eat fruit before exercising if you feel the need for some food before exerting yourself physically.

Take a thirty-to-sixty minute brisk aerobic walk, following the guidelines outlined in Step 5. Where possible, spend ten minutes standing or walking barefoot on a natural surface, connected to the earth.

At the end of your walk, practice the recommended stretching routine, available on the www.StressPandemic.com website.

On completion of your exercise routine, juice the produce that you prepared and drink it fresh.

Eat your full breakfast. Breakfast may consist of fruit, such as banana and berries; natural cereal such as organic oatmeal or brown rice (only cereals with no added sugar or artificial ingredients should be eaten); and nuts, such as almonds, walnuts, or Brazil nuts. Add pumpkin, flax, sunflower and other seeds if you like.

If you feel the need for added protein in your breakfast, feel free to incorporate egg whites into your morning meal.

■ Lunch

For lunch, eat foods high in protein and vegetables, and incorporate complex carbohydrates such as legumes (which are also rich in protein), brown rice, or sweet potatoes. As with all meals, try to enjoy the dining experience. Refrain from eating on the run; sit down for your meal.

Enjoy a cup of decaffeinated green tea, perhaps after lunch. Throughout the day, continue to drink purified, room-temperature water.

Do your best to cease all demanding and stressful activity before dinner.

■ Dinner

Try to eat dinner close to six p.m. or seven p.m., rather than late at night. Eat some quality protein and vegetables, but try to avoid a high amount of carbohydrates; avoiding carbohydrates altogether at night can actually be very good for the rhythm of the body. This is also the most important time to be vigilant about avoiding caffeine and minimizing or, better yet, avoiding alcohol.

After dinner, refrain from activities that stimulate your adrenaline or cause tension. Do something you enjoy or find relaxing. Avoid computer screens.

Go to bed at a time that will allow you seven and a half hours of sleep or more, depending on your needs.

THE FINAL STEPS

The final two steps, 8 and 9, provide insight for your continual self-assessment and also serve to illuminate the frontiers of your ongoing progress. These beacons will always be available to point you in the right direction.

STEP 8 : The Power of Awareness

- Practice the first seven steps and commit to them fully.
- Be mindful of your thoughts, your desires, and their likely consequences. Have an awareness of your lifestyle.
- Put your growing awareness of your innermost feelings, your thoughts, and your desires to good use by saying No to thoughts that don't serve you and Yes to thoughts that are of benefit to you.
- As you discover more ease and health in your life, allow yourself to embrace the present moment, enjoying fully what life has to offer here and now.
- Notice when your awareness is unnecessarily on the past or the future and gently bring it back to this very moment.
- Become aware of what you are holding on to, and see if you can begin to forgive yourself—to love yourself.

Questions to ask yourself:

- Where are my thoughts leading me?
- Are my thoughts leading me in the direction of the dark side of life (further from contentment and true wellness) or toward the bright side of life (closer to contentment and true wellness)?

- Where is my awareness? Is it on the past, the future, or the present?
- Can I let go of the past and the future and experience contentment and excitement of life right here and now?

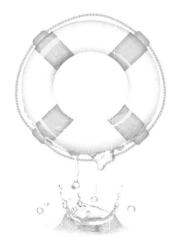

STEP 9 : Don't Give Up

- Remember that you have the power to move forward in your life, to fortify and empower yourself.
- Allow yourself time to break habits and form new ones.
- Understand that it is natural to stumble; the courage is in getting back up.
- Continue to pursue your application of the nine steps until you reach a thirty-day period of uninterrupted practice of the steps.
- Nurture your flame of hope and maintain your commitment, regardless of the challenges you encounter.

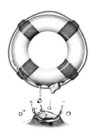

*Preparation and response
are the essence of the
Nine Natural Steps
to break the cycle of stress
and thrive.*PH

*For ongoing lifestyle awareness practices and support,
visit our health blog,
LIFERESTYLE™: www.LifeReStyle.org*

The Stress Pandemic is real,

Unchecked stress has very real consequences.

It can cause you pain and ultimately take your life.

*Take control of stress, before it takes control of you.*PH

Take pride in the scars on your skin,

to remember the adventures

*and places you have been.*_{PH}

PART THREE

SURVIVAL

My Story

Mens sana in corpore sano
(a healthy mind in a healthy body)
Juvenal

In 2010 I published the psychological thriller *Betrayal of Love and Freedom,* a novel that included a stylized account of my experiences with extreme stress and imbalance. I will not go into anywhere near as much detail here, but I would like to provide enough detail on the horror, struggle, and misery of my experience to serve as a deterrent and a warning to those who are at risk of prolonged, severe stress levels. I have sometimes reflected that if someone had explained to me the extreme danger of the way I was living—if they had honestly conveyed the misery of allowing myself to go over the edge by developing severe mind conditions and experiencing a nervous breakdown—I might have been able to avoid such a painful episode of my life.

I was, in fact, warned by friends who had suffered from mind conditions that I was under too much stress and it was showing, and they encouraged me to slow down. However, perhaps because of their own shame surrounding their experiences, they stopped short of explaining to me just how serious the situation was and what the potential outcome could be. Later, when I was institutionalized at the Menninger Clinic, I was made aware of the "golden rule": Never disclose your condition or your diagnosis of mental illness to anyone. This was intended as a protective measure against those (who are many, I discovered) who would manipulate a history of mental illness against a person. Because the stigma of mental illness is one of the biggest difficulties faced in recovering from it, we were told in no uncertain terms that we must adhere to the golden rule without fail. I considered the advice carefully, but I decided that regardless of the risks, I couldn't keep my experience to myself. I had to share the horrors of unchecked stress with everyone whom I thought it might help, in order to spread awareness and prevent others from going anywhere near where I went. How else can the cycle of misery be stopped, I thought to myself, if we don't have the courage to warn people of the misery we've experienced ourselves? I made the decision to break the golden rule.

It is my hope that by sharing my story I can help to prevent others from going anywhere near the edge. By demonstrating the results of unchecked stress and the pain of such an ordeal, as well as shining light on some of the warning signs, I hope that others who are at risk of heading in the same direction as I did will avert such a disaster. It is also my hope that people who have friends and loved ones suffering from severe stress or mind conditions can learn something from my account. We often find it difficult to understand the pain of someone struggling with a mind condition, because the affliction is not visible in the same way that a broken leg is. Greater awareness of mental illness is necessary in our society. Last, I hope that those who are currently suffering from mind conditions can benefit from my story by seeing that there is, in fact, a way to move forward and to once again be free.

In the beginning

I was a very lucky infant; I came into this world deeply loved. Given the number of infants who come into this world under the unfortunate circumstances of being unloved, unwanted, and abandoned, I had a huge head start in life. However, in an almost eerie prediction of things to come, I was branded for life at the age of two and a half years after spilling a boiling kettle of water on myself, which resulted in my hospitalization and a skin graft. This physical scar, though barely noticeable now, would be with me for the rest of my life. Much later, I would experience a very different form of branding that would turn my life upside down.

Born in the city of Auckland, New Zealand, I was the middle son of three boys. I was constantly in trouble and seemingly accident prone. My mother sometimes said that she thought I might never reach the age of twenty-one. As a young boy I was a sociable chatterbox and often the life of the party, easily finding much in the world to love. I often shared my sweets with everyone, to the point of having none left over for myself, but over time I would eventually notice that even with my natural tendency toward loyalty, caring for, and loving people, the same affection was not always returned.

When I was seven years old, my father promised me a red bicycle if I could perform six chin-ups. I was determined and practiced very hard to win this bike, eventually fulfilling my father's challenge and earning the longed-for bike. It was an old bike that was repainted in red and lacking some of the newer features I had seen elsewhere. Although it wasn't everything I had hoped for, I came to love it so very much, and it became my companion and a means of feeling free outside of the drama that often surrounded me in the rest of my life. I cycled around daydreaming, feeling free as a bird, until one day, living up to my accident-prone history, I had a head-on collision with an oncoming car. I somersaulted into the air and landed, head-first, on the hood of the car. My beloved bike was never to be replaced. I was very lucky to survive.

Although I have many fond memories of my childhood, my home life was not always easy or happy, as is the case for many of us. Much of my childhood coincided with a period of deep pain and sorrow for my mother, and this affected me greatly. Family life was often turbulent, and I witnessed a great deal of unhappiness. With the love a child can feel for his parents, it can be natural for the child to want his parents to live in a continual state of happiness. We know as adults, though, that no one can expect their expectations to be fulfilled all the time. It is up to us to fight for and earn what we desire and to work hard toward our ambitions and goals.

This was a philosophy instilled in me as a child by my father, with the ethics of hard work becoming ingrained in my outlook. This led to a great sense of pride and joy in whatever I achieved. My father loved us deeply and taught me much about the world. From my mother, I learned about love and forgiveness; she had a seemingly endless capacity for both.

Looking back now, I can see that my quest to attain material wealth began when I was eleven. At this time, my beloved dog died, the very same day as President Kennedy. I'd been nearing the bottom of my class, and I recall the teacher telling me once, as he held up my hand to give me a good strapping, "Huljich, one day you'll end up sweeping the streets." At the same time, I realized that I could no longer hide my school reports. I had to learn how to read and score higher marks. It began to appear to me quite clearly that money brought happiness because it gave one so many choices. I had witnessed my mother's distress at times when her finances were tight; I had seen others in difficult circumstances because of financial strain; and I had seen how much easier life was when money wasn't a problem. It seemed like such a simple, obvious solution.

It would take a long time for me to recognize the error of viewing financial freedom as the gateway to happiness. I was motivated to earn my own money so that I could enjoy freedom and share this freedom with others. I wanted to one day have my own family and fill our lives with joy and abundance; I wanted an environment for my family that would be comfortable and stable, where money was never an issue. I saw it as the key to the life I wanted and the escape from the life I had. From that moment forward, I replaced being a rebel and enjoying time with friends with making money; I mowed lawns, collected bottles, caddied at the local golf club, and parked people's cars. Slowly, I watched my little bank account grow.

The best-laid plans

At age eleven, I formed my best-laid plans. I have vivid memories of cycling around the Auckland waterfront and dreaming of the beautiful home I would like to have one day. I wanted a big house, a flashy car, a boat, to travel the world, to be my own boss, and to do whatever I wanted. I wanted to eat my meals in restaurants, which, in those days (the 1960s), was a luxury reserved for only the rich and famous. Throughout my teenage years I developed into an ambitious young man. But was I following my innermost feelings and values, or was I choosing a path based on what I thought would amount to "success," and would that vision of success bring me the happiness I desired?

The impression I had of life was that money made the world go round. From a very early age, we're conditioned to value money almost more than anything else in life. Money is disguised in different ways. We're taught to equate money with security, success, and a sense of freedom. As a teenager, my best-laid plans emulated what my dad taught me: "Work hard, gain experience and knowledge, and become a success." As a result, I bought into the marketing of the lifestyle of the rich and famous promoted by the dawning age of advertising in the mid-sixties. This was the era of Elvis, the Beach Boys, the Beatles, and the seduction of Hollywood. Even though I grew up in a remote part of the world, I, too, bought into this myth of money. I wanted to reach the Emerald City at the end

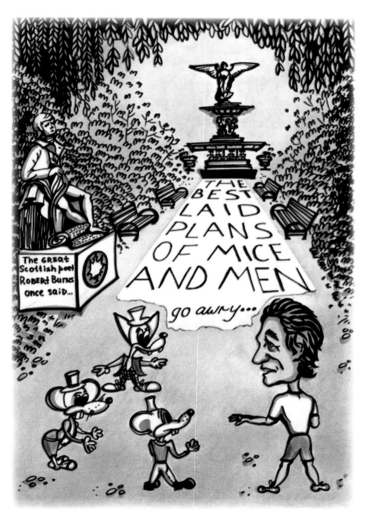

"The best laid schemes of mice and men oft go awry / And leave us nothing but grief and pain" – Robert Burns

of the Yellow Brick Road, and I wanted to win that pot of gold waiting for me at the end of the rainbow. As a young man, I confused monetary success with achieving peace of mind, contentment, and every happiness. My motivating ambition was to attain the freedom to live how I wanted to and, while doing so, to remain kind and generous to everyone in my life. I believed that by simply working hard, playing hard, and trying to keep out of trouble, I had a balance in life and was being true to myself. But boy, was I wrong!

Riding the tsunami

I continued working toward my goals throughout my high school years. During my time at university, I became ever more involved in my business career, so much so that I had to drop out of my degree program before completing it in order to tend to the enterprises I had been developing.

I had always been particular about the food I ate and had developed a special fascination with it. My mother and grandmother were excellent cooks, and I spent much time in the kitchen. After being involved in a variety of businesses as a young adult, I decided in the early 1980s to follow my passion for supporting the health of the body through natural and high-quality foods. For years I had felt that the typical Western diet was heading in the wrong direction. I knew we could do much better, and I was excited by the challenge of delivering a high-quality product to the market, one that would set new standards of excellence and be of benefit to people.

I observed how the foods we were eating were having increasingly catastrophic effects on both our health and on the planet. Genetic engineering was in its infancy. I had a strong desire to get involved in organic foods, even though at the time that category was still largely unknown. As a consumer, I believed that most of our foods were overprocessed and were produced in ways that showed little regard for our humanity or our planet. I wanted to make a difference for humanity. In time, my passion developed into a calling to invest in something with greater purpose. This led me to launch an organic and natural food company in 1985 named Best Corporation, of which I was cofounder, chairman, and joint-CEO. Its motto:

Good, Better, Best.
Never shall I rest.
Until my good is better,
*and my better best!*PH

I enjoyed trying to turn lemons into lemonade. The company began as I saw an opportunity in the pork products industry, an industry that suffered from overcapacity, a negative image, low profits, and diminishing growth. It was a challenge, but we took a unique approach to creating a superior, healthy, quality product that transformed the industry in New Zealand by setting new standards of excellence. That success opened the way for ventures into a variety of organic foods, such as organic meat, poultry, seafood, and vegetable products.

One of the most beautiful parts of the dream for me was the creation of the Best Corporation family. The success of the company was shared among all employees, and our culture was something I was extremely proud of. We had a policy of taking on unskilled workers, often struggling immigrants, training them to the highest standards, and then paying them well above the prevailing wage. The only requirement for such a position was enthusiasm. A committee was formed within Best to support employees in their lives, for example, by granting interest-free loans to those who were in difficult situations and were sometimes even victims of domestic violence seeking to escape and build a new life. In the end, these loans were all forgiven when we sold the company. Our executives were encouraged to take vacation time, and they were discouraged from working nights or weekends. Best became a flourishing family whose members took the utmost pride in their affiliation with the company and its community.

Pioneering and cultivating this dream was a huge challenge. To manifest and execute the vision required many long hours. The challenge of juggling family and business while not heeding my innermost feelings eventually caught up with me, even though part of me knew that something had to give. Unfortunately, that something turned out to be my health. Although I was still in touch with one aspect of my innermost feelings, I see now that my ambitions pushed me too far. My goals and my contentment were wildly diverging; a huge gulf between the two had developed. As much as I was doing my best to help those within my sphere of influence, I neglected myself. Later, during my time at the Menninger Clinic, I would come to realize that I was trying to take care of everyone except myself. In the end, I was the one who lost out.

Looking back now, I see that I had plenty of warnings.

The signs were everywhere. My marketing manager and friend, Chris Thornton, who was dying of cancer, confronted me, saying that I was neglecting myself. My longtime bank manager, David Brown, who told me that he, too, was dying of cancer, warned me that I was working too hard and needed to slow down. There were many others in my life who echoed this sentiment and begged me repeatedly to slow down. There was even a Japanese business leader who sensed that I was lost. He suggested that I take more time for myself, buy a winery, and take an interest in something other than business and my family. My father warned me to slow down; he even apologized for telling me to work so hard when I was growing up. When he bought me a set of golf clubs, Dad told me that my stress levels were out of control. He implored me to relax and slow down. He, at the age of sixty-one, was battling prostate cancer. Five years later, just before he died, he bought me a second set of golf clubs. "Son, you need to slow down," he said. "What is it that you want to achieve?" He pleaded with me to play golf, but I never did. I never found the time.

I needed to take sleeping tablets in order to sleep. My circadian rhythms were badly out of kilter due to increased global travel for business, spanning multiple time zones. Even family holidays, which usually saw me simply working from a different location, contributed to this downward spiral. I had to visit a dentist many times for chronic grinding of my teeth during sleep due to the pressure I was under; I was given a mouth guard and told not to worry. Ultimately, I began to question where I was in life. It seemed that the sense of wonder and happiness I'd had when I was young was now somehow missing. Indeed, anything resembling that youthful jubilance seemed distant, as if it had occurred in another life altogether.

Ironically, around this time I reached a point, when I was in my forties, where I had achieved what some might see as the ideal, successful life. I was living in a newly built, 30,000-square-foot home that I had designed for my wife, my three sons, and myself, which had an outdoor swimming pool, a twenty-five-meter indoor swimming pool with a domed roof, fifteen bathrooms, a tennis court, a squash court, and a croquet lawn, all set amid lush gardens and palm trees. I owned a Porsche, a Ferrari, and a yacht. We vacationed in luxurious locations around the world. I had realized my dream of building a successful food company and producing something that I believed in, all while being my own boss. However, the first effects of prolonged, extreme stress had begun to manifest, and little did I know that these symptoms were only the tip of the iceberg.

Life is a series of waves; we're all riding one wave or another at any given time. The more we polish and wax our surfboard, learn about the rhythm of the wave, and develop our stamina, the more we tend to relish the challenge of life and get high from the thrill of riding ever bigger waves. As a great challenger in life, I wanted more. *Can I do more? Can I experience more? Can I have more?* These were the questions I asked myself. I was constantly testing and challenging my boundaries of knowledge, experience, and courage. I hadn't realized that what I had thought of as the perfect wave—this trajectory that I had been following for many years—might be morphing into something more dangerous. It had grown steadily until, one day, it would reveal itself as a tsunami.

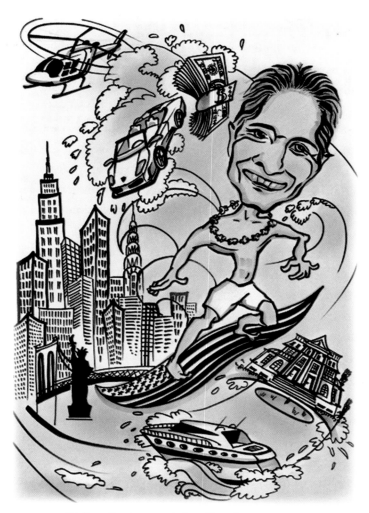

Riding the tsunami; heading for a wipeout

Heading toward the edge

I had been aware of a strange, abiding feeling for years—a sense of dread combined with emptiness. It would abate momentarily when something truly wonderful happened, but this would be only a short respite from what I later came to understand was depression. I became aware that there was something wrong with me. It wasn't a physical ailment but an emotional and mental one.

Regardless of any success I achieved, the resulting sense of satisfaction or joy proved fleeting at best, always leaving me feeling despondent and wanting more. Although I experienced moments of peace, happiness, and contentment, they were short-lived and soon overcome by anxiety and a dull, flat feeling in my chest and stomach. I was unable to discern why I was feeling the way I did but knew somewhere that it was a form of depression.

It felt as though I was sinking into the quicksand of myself, and the more I struggled against myself, the deeper I sank, down and down into a dark hole within, from which there was no escape. I was losing my grip on reality.

What was happening to me was actually occurring physiologically, within my body. The neurochemistry of my brain was becoming more disrupted every day. My wife begged me to take a hearing test, as she felt that I wasn't listening to her anymore. She was right, but the real reason why I wasn't listening was because I didn't have any time to myself. My waking hours from morning until night were occupied with meetings and responding to needs and expectations of others. I resorted to writing notes to myself in the middle of the night with a flashlight pen and pad I kept next to my bed.

My time was devoted not only to my family but also to my stockholders, and I took this professional responsibility very seriously. When we had publicly listed Best Corporation, the new, public stockholders were welcomed into the company to join in the adventure of Best's journey. My two brothers and I, the original owners and still the majority shareholders, ensured that the status of the public stockholders was equal to ours. We never paid any of our expenses through the company, instead paying for all costs incurred out of pocket; we traveled only in economy class for all our flights, despite the prosperity of the company; and we took no salary from the company, paying ourselves only a symbolic one dollar per day. Although this information was not made public until after we sold our shares to a multinational corporation two years later, we did this because we felt a binding moral obligation to all investors. We chose to be rewarded on the same basis as all other stockholders—that is, to be rewarded only through appreciation of company stock value and by dividends. This sense of responsibility to the company and investors led to great sadness for me when my father was dying, because I found it difficult to spend the time I wanted to with him.

My brothers and I also established a foundation for children, a charity that provided opportunities for terminally ill children to enjoy a dream vacation with their family. Again, we refused to make the one-million-dollar founding contribution through the company's accounts to lower our tax bill and instead donated the money from our personal finances. We did the same when donating anonymously to other worthy causes.

It was at this time, after a six-year struggle with cancer, that my father passed away. Despite my work obligations, I managed to visit him every day unless I was traveling for business, but it was never enough; I longed to spend much more time with him, and it always seemed that business was cutting short our visits. It was after my father's passing that we decided to sell Best Corporation. His death had a profound effect on me. My depression was escalating, and I was unable to cope. My father's passing was the final straw, and it thrust me into a deep state of inconsolable grief, unleashing an avalanche of unstoppable anxiety.

I went to see a psychiatrist recommended to me by Dr. Tony Antunovich, my general practitioner of many years. The psychiatrist prescribed medication for my anxiety, but by this stage, it was too late; I was already fading. Aside from grinding my teeth, experiencing anxiety, and taking sleeping tablets, my depression was growing stronger. I had become a runaway train hurtling toward a precipice at breakneck speed, unable to come to a halt. The depression I had been experiencing became severe.

One morning I awoke in the fetal position. I was scared and cold and the only way to warm my body was to take a warm bath. I was shaking and shivering. I felt afraid of anything and everything in the world—every passing shadow—and found comfort only in the darkness of my room, hiding from the outside world. I was incapable of making any decisions on my own, from what to wear to what to eat. I wanted only to take

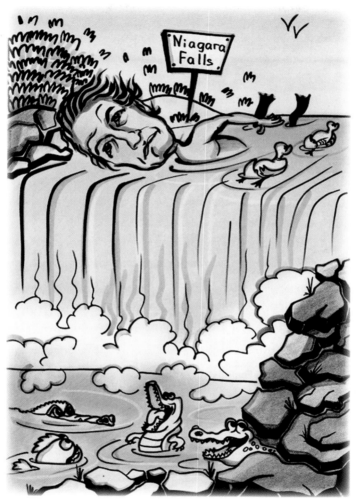

Unheeded warnings—heading toward the edge

a sleeping pill so I could escape to the dark from the agony of consciousness. I remember wondering, *Would anyone be able to understand what I'm going through?* I understood that I had probably been suffering from mild depression for a number of years without realizing it.

After I spent three days bedridden with exhaustion and unable to face the world, my wife and I visited my psychiatrist, who warned me of the seriousness of the situation—that I had developed severe depression. She warned that I had to exercise extreme caution and banish all stress from my life, as my health was in grave danger after years of accumulated stress and exhaustion. She prescribed stronger medication, this time lithium, in addition to the antianxiety medication I had been prescribed before. At first, the darkness of the depression lifted. However, my condition continued to deteriorate, and I soon developed severe mood swings, ranging from paranoia and deep depression to euphoria and a sense of invincibility. I was clearly not "me" during the extremes of these mood swings, and my behavior would be irrational and completely at odds with the Paul people knew. I wouldn't know why, after a mood swing, I had acted in ways that I would ordinarily never want to act. This pattern continued for months, and there was nothing I could do—no amount of vacationing, pleasure, or attempted relaxation could alleviate the problem. My psychiatrist's response was to increase my dosage of medication every month until I was near the maximum allowable dosage.

The day I lost love and freedom

My condition deteriorated steadily for a number of months until, one week, things began going dreadfully wrong with my body and mind.

The mood swings I was experiencing had become extremely volatile in the week leading up to my breakdown. One day, my eldest son, who was nineteen at the time, wanted to take me out to lunch, probably as an attempt to cheer me up, as it was becoming obvious that something wasn't right with me. People in the restaurant, too, noticed that there was something wrong with me. For days, my eyes had been glazed, lit up, as if I were on hyperalert or high on drugs, and it was clear that the restaurant patrons were unsettled by my appearance. I couldn't pay attention to anything my son said for more than a few seconds, and I was having difficulty understanding his words. Then, out of nowhere, I suddenly couldn't speak. I remember vaguely hearing a question that my son had asked me, opening my mouth to respond, and then nothing coming out. I was actually unable to get my body to perform a normally effortless task—producing sound. I sat there, motionless, shocked at what was happening to me and unable to do anything about it. Watching myself from the inside, willing myself to speak, I was terrified to realize that for the first time in my memory I was not in control of my body. I was later to understand that my neurochemistry had gone haywire, and my brain simply could not, or would not, make this connection.

My behavior soon became so outrageous that, on one occasion, I snatched a cell phone out of an executive's hand and threw it into my swimming pool, annoyed at the disturbance of it ringing after I had already asked him to turn it off. There was another business meeting at which I ended up taking off all my clothes, right on down to my underwear, in front of all my executives and board members.

In the days leading up to my breakdown, I had taken to jumping off dangerously high walls around the grounds of our home. I was perhaps convinced that I could fly, but instead I would end up hurting myself. My wife was horrified whenever she saw the evidence of it on my bloodied feet.

Very soon, I experienced a complete mental breakdown. I can't begin to describe the horror of that day, but luckily no one was physically hurt. Although there are large portions of the day that I have never been able to recall, and frankly, I haven't especially wanted to, I do remember an entire episode at a gas station on the morning of the breakdown. My two brothers, along with two executives, had taken me out for a drive, hoping it would relax me. At the gas station near our house, I pulled out my wallet and started trying to hand out hundred-dollar bills to whomever would take them, while my brother and business colleagues had to force me back into the car for my own good. When we eventually reached home, by which time several family members and family friends had appeared to help in the growing crisis, I demanded that everyone form a circle around me as I went around, one by one, telling people of their flaws and my personal grievances with them. Perhaps luckily for me, I can't actually remember anything I said, but I'm sure it would be further humiliating for me if I did. I then began hallucinating that I was Jesus Christ and could walk on water as I waded in our fountain, making the sign of a crucifix with my hands.

By the early afternoon, it was clear to the family members who had gathered at my home to avert disaster that I had lost it. A mental health crisis team was immediately called to my home. I was declared mentally unsound and lost my rights as a New Zealand citizen: I had to surrender my passport, any contracts I entered into were null and void, I was prohibited from accessing my bank accounts, and all my credit cards were confiscated. I was now considered a ward of the state, under the guardianship of the government and only spared from immediate institutionalization on the basis of a probation arrangement made with the crisis team. The crisis team's head psychiatrist diagnosed my condition as bipolar disorder, a diagnosis that ten other psychiatrists would confirm during the following months. Everyone was afraid; no one understood what bipolar disorder was. It was a taboo subject, and a decision was made to keep my condition absolutely secret.

Sitting on my bed and hiding from my life, I felt that everything I treasured most in life had vanished. I'd just been stripped of my freedom. What made this even worse was that when I turned to find reassurance in the eyes of those I loved most, I only sensed their fear and terror at what I'd become. In my mind, I had lost the two most valuable forces in my life: love and freedom.

What love and freedom have I now? Imprisoned physically in my own home, against my will, I'm a prisoner of my own mind. Thoughts such as these constantly raced through my head.

I have been given pills. They say I must take them to stabilize the chemical imbalance in my brain, and so I do; but with every waking minute, I can feel the drugs taking control of my every movement—every aspect, every feeling, and every breath I take—all while under twenty-four-hour surveillance. I feel like a man condemned to be hanged, who confesses all his wrongdoings in a desperate plea to be spared. I'm so confused. Is it the drugs? Or is it the guilt because I humiliated and embarrassed everyone I love? To think that I made a fool of myself in front of all those people... my sons, my wife, my mother and family, my colleagues, friends, and even strangers. This is agony.

Where, oh where, and how and when did I cross the line? And where were the rock-solid warning signs that I was a danger to myself, those around me, and society in general? When did I become an embarrassment to almost everyone I know in life, including myself? I saw the terror in my wife and children's eyes when they looked at my bloody feet. Shit, what happened to me? Maybe I have no choice but to just accept it and give in. How low can I go before my spirit is totally crushed? Where is my spirit right now? Did it desert me or did I desert it? Which came first? Am I merely operating off the flicker of a flame right now? Why couldn't the doctors stop this before I got to where I am now? They should have warned me of the consequences.

Why me? Why did it have to happen now?

The search for a cure

In time, my condition stabilized with the help of medication and strict supervision, including the presence of a nurse twenty-four hours a day. The extreme mood swings I had been experiencing—the most obvious symptoms of bipolar disorder—abated, and I regained my rights as a citizen. I was told in no uncertain terms that I had bipolar disorder, that there was no cure for this disorder, and that I would need to be on medication for the rest of my life. While medication could help prevent severe mood swings, I was still patently aware of the emptiness, depression, and lifelessness of my condition.

I knew that I wasn't myself, that I wasn't the true Paul. I had lost touch with my spirit and was totally dependent on medication. Determined to free myself from the shackles of bipolar disorder, I traveled with the help of my wife, mother, and brothers to the world-renowned Mayo Clinic in Rochester, Minnesota, where heads of state traveled from around the world to receive expert medical care. After undergoing many tests over a period of twelve days and meeting with the head of the psychiatric department, I was told again that I had bipolar disorder, that there was no cure, and that I would be dependent on drugs for the rest of my life. I would need to be very careful about my lifestyle and the amount of stress I might take on, he cautioned. I was also told that my condition was the result of prolonged stress—both emotional and in the realm of work—although it was also common to hear people talk about causes of mental imbalance being hereditary or genetic. I disagree with this reasoning, believing instead in the model of learned behavior, on the basis of my own experience and research. The prevalence of attributing mind conditions to genetics concerns me because of its tendency to convince people that they are powerless. It can lead to people feeling that they are without choice, while potentially promoting complacency and encouraging the "easy way out" of giving up on the commitment to true recovery. However, it is my view that, regardless of whether or not there is a genetic link, mind conditions are ultimately triggered by the way we live our lives. It is the psychological stress that we endure in our lives that eventually leads to the onset of a mind condition. Whether or not some individuals are more genetically predisposed to mind conditions than others, we still possess the power of choice in how we live our lives. I often respond to proponents of the hereditary theory that my ability to cure myself is proof that, genetic or not, we ultimately have control.

I was not satisfied with the answers I was given. I could not accept that there was no cure for my condition; I was convinced that there must be some way for me to rediscover my true self and break free of the "chemical straitjacket" (as I often referred to the reliance on psychotropic medication) that had imprisoned me. I asked for the Mayo Clinic's doctors' advice on what more I could do to expand my knowledge and understanding of depression, anxiety, addictions, and bipolar disorder. They directed me to the Menninger Clinic in Topeka, Kansas.

The Menninger Clinic was a serious institution. I was required to sign away my rights (after having regained them from the New Zealand government only weeks earlier) and place myself at the mercy of the clinic's doctors in order to be admitted as a patient. After much consideration, I submitted to their requirements, signing away any power of mine, my wife's, or my family's, to discharge me from the institution. The only way I was going to leave was if and when the doctors decided I was ready to leave.

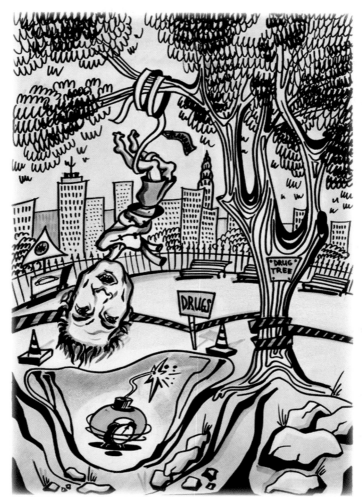

Only a matter of time

Time bomb

I had been told that I was a time bomb—that the more pronounced effects of my condition would, eventually, reassert themselves, and I would experience another full breakdown. I already felt branded for life with the stigma of being "mentally ill." The pain of hurting the people I loved most with my failure to be the "real Paul," and the alleged certainty of another breakdown, was more than I could bear. I needed to understand as much as possible about my condition if I was going to beat it, and the Menninger Clinic, I was told, was the next step.

I spent six weeks in the clinic. The first week was immensely challenging, and I begged the doctors to release me so that I could return to my family, but they refused. I eventually accepted that I had much to learn about my condition and that I was in the right place for doing so. In time, I came to embrace all that the clinic had to offer, learning everything I could from official channels and also from speaking with numerous other patients about their experiences. I seized every available opportunity to further my understanding of stress and mental illness—attending classes on anger, grief, guilt, and addictions, among others, even though some did not apply to me.

After studying mental illness from a number of angles, it became apparent that full recovery was elusive for most. It seemed that the clinic had a revolving door, with patients returning again and again to recover from breakdowns and relapses. In the end, I gained the confidence of the doctors and was released, having a much more comprehensive understanding of my condition, but even with such expanded knowledge, I had to admit that I didn't have all the answers, let alone a cure. Still, I was more determined than ever to reclaim my power and my life.

I also began to understand that the clinic's revolving door was a result of the inability of patients to withstand the stress of their lives in the real world. While many could achieve a partial recovery within the protective boundaries of the clinic, they found the demands and challenges of their everyday lives too much to handle. Eventually, they would relapse and return to the clinic. I recognized that, in order to be free of my condition, I would need to conquer stress. This was in addition to the advice of the doctors—that in order to lead anything resembling a normal life, I would need to keep my stress under control. I knew that I needed to learn how to master stress.

Rebuilding myself

Upon returning to New Zealand, I saw the causes of my condition in a new light. I could recognize a variety of factors that caused emotional stress and pain for many years, as well as the stress and demands I had been dealing with in business. These had been brought to my attention at different times, and I had noticed them myself. However, the one understanding that made all the difference was to recognize that it was the "old me," the "old Paul," who got me into this mess. This meant accepting that, if I wanted to live fully again and beat my condition, I had to change myself. I had to be proactive in stripping myself right back to the core of who I was and rebuilding myself from there. I had to create a new Paul—one who wouldn't make himself sick and who would be able to experience life in its full wonder.

I had met many patients in the Menninger Clinic with histories of substance abuse as a means for coping with stress. The approach advocated by Alcoholics Anonymous was widely respected and praised in this area. However, I felt that I had to go a step further than this approach. While AA was able to support people in recovering and breaking through their addictions, part of its approach was based on participants never touching drink, or the substance, again. While this made sense because of the toxic nature of alcohol and drugs, I felt that what I was aiming for was slightly different: I wanted to be able to withstand the pressures of life again. I wanted to be strong enough to live life fully, with all its ups and downs, so that I wouldn't have to insulate myself from life the way I had been since my breakdown. I speculated that, if I could cleanse myself of my harmful psychological tendencies and rebuild myself both physically and psychologically, then I should be able to take any form of stress and deal with life's challenges without having to shield myself. Although the doctors had been adamant about accepting my condition and accepting that I would be dependent on drugs for the rest of my life, as well as needing to keep stress to a minimum, I refused to believe that this was the only way. I knew that it was possible for me to live a full life again.

Through trial and error, through my research into all facets of health, and through interviewing and speaking with whomever I could find to talk to about health, I began developing processes that would correct the chemical imbalance in my brain that doctors had told me I was suffering from as a result of prolonged stress. I realized that many parts of the person I had become, as well as any addictions or obsessions that I had, were formed by habit. I came to understand that many habits are formed over a thirty-day period of repetition and that these habits shape our lives. To deprogram my body and mind of harmful habits, I had to be disciplined about aiming for thirty consecutive days of overriding old habits with new ones. Like a child learning to walk, I had to start from the beginning.

I studied nutrition with the aim of supporting the brain's neurochemical balance, and I completely overhauled my diet. With the help of extensive research and my own experimentation, I was able to ensure that my body was being nourished for optimal health. I studied different forms of exercise and their effects on the body, designing and implementing an exercise program that I gradually increased and refined to a point where my body was receiving maximal benefits. I wanted to be in optimum health and was inspired by the image of a perfectly cut diamond, with fifty-eight facets in ideal proportions. If any one detail of such a diamond is compromised, the brilliance of the gem will be lost. It was the same with my own self—every aspect had to be in perfect balance.

After studying numerous practices, I developed my own meditation processes, making use of powerful affirmations, and implemented other stress-reduction techniques that I would practice daily. In time, I focused on changing my thinking. I remembered visiting the ruins of the healing temple used by ancient Greek doctors and how inspired I was by the methods they employed. I used this approach as a starting point to reprogram how I felt about the past and the future and to appreciate how beautiful it is to enjoy life in the present moment.

Beyond my commitment to rebuilding myself, I also wanted to live in balance and ensure that my way of life was practical, so I tailored the bulk of my wellness regimen to a program that I could follow every morning, even when traveling. I knew that the morning often was the only part of the day when I could devote the necessary amount of time to my well-being. I wanted my routine to be as basic and natural as possible; I wanted a system that was easy to implement and required a minimum of equipment.

As I slowly crafted and implemented the new steps in my life, I found that with a little bit of patience, my attitude began to change. I started to feel better. I started to realize that simplicity was powerful. For instance, seeing food in terms of natural and unnatural, processed and unprocessed, made supporting my health a relatively simple matter.

I continued to remind myself that the "old me" was the cause of my sickness, and therefore it was my responsibility to build a "new me." I knew that I was going to be challenged by my habits, and indeed I was; it took perseverance, focus, and patience to gradually rebuild myself into a new, healthy person. Many of the habits I had formed in my prior life had an addictive quality to them, and I came to see that I had used them as crutches to be able to cope with stress, because they temporarily made me feel better. I had to find the courage to say no to my habits and to other unhealthy demands in my life and instead learn to follow my innermost feelings.

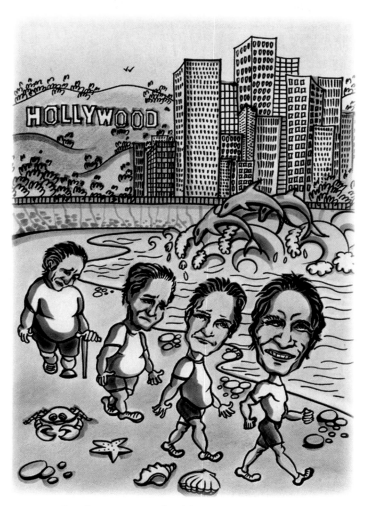

It takes time to rebuild or ReStyle your life.

This period of transformation was hugely challenging. I would sometimes liken myself to someone who was recovering from a stroke, who had to relearn basic motor skills. Similarly, I felt that I had to learn to walk again, one step at a time. I knew that I had to fight back; I had to be proactive. I reminded myself that it was OK if I fell over time and time again, as long as I kept chipping away as if I were making a hole in a huge dam; it would take time, but eventually I would break through.

I was also dealt a severe blow during this time of recovery, in what was the saddest period of my life. I had been informed, while at the Menninger Clinic, that 80 percent of marriages failed following a nervous breakdown by one of the partners. I was determined to ensure that my marriage was part of the 20 percent that would emerge from a nervous breakdown intact. Indeed, preserving my marriage—along with the welfare of my children—was the primary motivator in my determination to recover from my breakdown.

However, as my recovery progressed, I became painfully aware of the toll that the stress and upheaval of the preceding few years had taken on my wife and on our relationship. My exhaustion as a result of my dedication to business, as well as the emotional turmoil of the lead-up to my breakdown and its aftermath, had resulted in a strained relationship. Both my wife and I did our best over many months to address her understandable hurt and anger. We worked with two different marriage counselors. Both of us were desperate to repair our broken relationship and to bridge the gulf between us, but the pressure of the recent years and the breakdown had wreaked irreparable damage on our marriage.

I experienced a sense of being at a breaking point. It eventually became frighteningly clear to me that if I didn't leave home, I would not be able to become the new Paul that I knew I had to grow into in order to survive. I knew, somewhere inside, that if I didn't rebuild myself and make changes in my life to move through the constant pain of our relationship, I would soon be hit with one of the "big four": another nervous breakdown, cancer, a heart attack, or a stroke. This was the biggest shock and most painful disappointment of my life, but the imperative to leave home came from the knowledge that I would be of more use to those I loved if I were alive rather than dead. If I wanted to be there for my three sons and for my wife and those who needed me, I had to make my survival the priority, no matter how gut-wrenching the implications were. I understood that, in order to survive, I had to leave home and leave the people I loved most.

This move to leave home was not only the saddest episode of my life but also the most stressful. I was afraid that the shock and trauma of it would push me over the edge and trigger another nervous breakdown. I had been rebuilding myself for nine months at the time, and I was frightened that I was not going to be able to handle the transition. I repeatedly asked my mother to tell me if she noticed any significant changes in my behavior. I increased the amount of time I devoted to my regimen of the nine steps and worked hard in dealing with the pain of leaving my family. I was working hard during the day at business, trying to keep myself focused on something other than the sadness of what was happening. But there were always times where the darkness would find a way in; it seemed to follow me, and whenever I wasn't working or trying to stay occupied with other family members or friends, it would stalk me in my hotel room. Even when I was keeping my mind occupied, it would slip back into dwelling on the pain that was my constant companion. Habits that I had conquered in the months of rebuilding myself before I left home would return, and I sometimes would find myself tempted to seek escape in having a drink or eating junk food, though I was able to remain free of these habits for the most part. My loneliness would, at times, overwhelm me, and the guilt and shame I felt weighed heavily on me. Despite the immense challenges of this period, I was able to continue my focus on the nine steps and eventually move through this pain and continue my journey to true wellness. I saw my children regularly, and eventually, after a year or two, my former wife and I began to develop a healthy friendship whereby we could continue to share in the lives of our sons together.

Fighting back

At first I felt a little like a man with a walking stick, but in time, I grew stronger, able to stand taller and leave my crutch behind. In time, with tremendous focus and determination, I changed. Not only did I improve physically but also emotionally. My whole outlook on life began to change, and I kept improving in every way. Eventually, I reached a stage where I felt something inside that I hadn't known since childhood: a wonderful sense of contentment and peace. No matter what was happening in my life, no matter what the challenge was, I had a feeling of resilience and being able to bounce back.

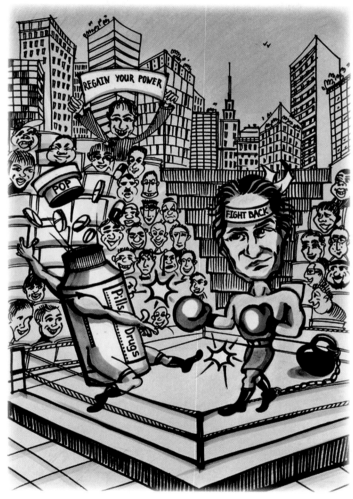

Fight back and win.

The challenges were endless: ever since my return from the Menninger Clinic, I had resumed my involvement in business. Early on, just a month or two after returning to New Zealand, I had flown with several members of my team to Japan to work on a deal on which millions of dollars had already been spent for research. On the way back, however, I noticed that my hands were shaking; something was not right, and my body was making it known. I took it as a warning that I had to be conscious of balancing my work life with my new commitment to my health and recovery, and despite the pressures of business and a sense of obligation to those I was working with, I found the courage to say No to demands that I knew were not in harmony with my best interests. The challenges in my business dealings and my separation from my wife and eventual divorce posed huge difficulties for me. Perhaps the greatest source of distress was the ongoing friction I experienced with my older brother and his family, dating back to well before my breakdown, due to a number of deep-rooted issues. Throughout it all, I was committed to making time each day, despite the demands of my life, to devote to practicing the nine steps.

As I became the "new me," challenges didn't keep me down for long, as they had in the past. I realized that the feelings that were now returning to me were something I had only experienced in the distant past; possibly many of us have this contentment early in our lives if we are lucky, but then we forget that it ever existed. Just like a person who develops a painful condition and lives with it for many years, eventually coming to accept the pain as normal, we can too easily come to accept our stress and disharmony as normal, when in truth, contentment and happiness are possible. The more I experienced this natural high of inner strength, wellness, and peace, the more I valued it and wanted to preserve it.

I had rebuilt my life to a large extent, developing new business projects and addressing issues with earlier businesses, structures, and relationships. Still, I knew there was one final hurdle to clear: I had to free myself from reliance on medication for bipolar disorder. I had been told I was a time bomb waiting to go off; I was still being monitored by monthly blood tests with my psychiatrist, and I seemed always to be on the defensive and looked upon with doubt. It was clear that I was answerable to the psychiatrist and that I would be required to appear for immediate assessment if ever he received a complaint or expression of doubt from someone. I knew I would never be free until I was off the medication. A memory from my childhood often came to mind: my grandfather, an expert stonemason, was asked by our neighbor to break down an enormous boulder on his property that had become a hindrance and could not be moved. I remember watching this slight man, standing only five feet two inches tall, carefully examining the massive rock, feeling the surface with his hand, his steely eyes intent on his goal. He determined the weak spot and then, with a single blow from his sledgehammer, this finely built man shattered the boulder into pieces. This simple, potent image stayed with me. Despite the magnitude of the task that lay ahead of me, I would use my focus and my wisdom to come off the drugs.

After eighteen months of concerted effort with the nine steps, I felt ready to free myself of dependence on medication. I had been under the supervision of a psychiatrist in my hometown of Auckland ever since my return from the Menninger Clinic. One day, I asked him if he would support me in coming off the medication I was taking for bipolar disorder. With his supervision, as well as the watchful eyes of family and friends, my dosage was gradually dropped. Naturally, I was nervous. Every doctor had told me I would need to be medicated for the rest of my life. If there was any indication that something was not right in my behavior or mood, I would have to return to the medication.

Over a period of months my medication intake was slowly decreased, until, with my psychiatrist's blessing, I was finally free of the drugs. Even I was surprised to see that I had remained stable, and I felt better than I could ever remember. However, there was still one final step to knowing that I had completed a full recovery from bipolar disorder: I had to be tested in the coliseum of life. I felt like a battle scarred warrior.

I have to say that, in the past 14 years since I've been medication-free, the stress in my life has been more intense than ever before. It has been a time of enormous upheaval and change, and at times I must admit that I was nervous that the stress would push me back over the edge. However, through it all, I have felt continuously grounded and grateful for my life, always experiencing a sense of contentment, to varying degrees, and joy to be alive.

For more than twelve years, I have been completely free of any psychotropic medication, including sleeping tablets. I have had no need for a therapist or psychiatrist and have had no relapses whatsoever of bipolar disorder, depression, or any other psychological condition or imbalance.

Although I don't recommend leading a stressful life, I have found that by maintaining the Nine Natural Steps that I developed during my period of rebuilding and remaining committed to their principles, I have been able to deal with more stress than I ever had previously. At the same time, the fleeting moments of happiness I once experienced have grown into a sustained state of contentment. Furthermore, I enjoy the best health I have ever experienced, and I am often told I look far younger than my years.

These nine steps are my approach for managing stress in one's life. Doctors informed me that the only chance I had of leading something akin to a normal life was to manage my stress. I soon came to the realization that if I wanted to truly free myself from what I had been told was an unbeatable condition, I would need to go further than managing stress—I would need to master it. The Nine Natural Steps enabled me to cure myself of all components of my depression and bipolar disorder and to master the underlying cause of these imbalances: stress. It was my success in beating stress that allowed me to do the "impossible" and free myself from serious mind conditions.

We are all challenged in life, and we are all betrayed. The lesson to be learned in our lives is the ability to love and, most important, to be able to love ourselves. We must learn to forgive ourselves for the mistakes we have made; we must learn to find that wonderful place of joy, fulfillment, and contentment within. I strongly believe that people have much to gain by practicing the Nine Natural Steps and implementing them in some way or another. I wish you every success in the coliseum of life.

DOCTOR'S DECLARATION

TONY ANTUNOVICH declares as follows:

1. I am a medical doctor in general practice licensed to practice medicine in New Zealand. I am fully familiar with the facts and circumstances herein, and I submit this declaration. I could and would competently testify to the matters stated herein.
2. Paul Huljich has been a patient of mine for the past twenty years and attends regularly for medical check-ups and good health maintenance. In mid-1997 he developed symptoms of a Major Depressive Disorder, and was treated for this with antidepressant medication. He later was diagnosed with Bipolar Disorder, and treated for this with further mood-stabilizing medications. His lowest point was March 1998, when he suffered a complete mental breakdown. He ceased all psychotropic medication towards the end of 1999, and has remained well since.
3. Indeed, since that time, Mr. Huljich has been in great health. Apart from regularly taking the medication Propecia for his hair loss, and the occasional course of antibiotics for Upper Respiratory Tract infection, he has not been prescribed any other medication – specifically, no anti-anxiety, no anti-depressant, no sedative/hypnotic and no anti-psychotic medication. Further, Mr. Huljich has not been hospitalized for any reason over the past twelve years, and neither has he been seen by any other practitioner for any mental illness.
4. In sum, Mr. Huljich is of sound mind and judgment, and has clearly been so since at least the year 2000.

I declare under penalty of perjury, under the laws of the United States of America, that the foregoing is true and correct.

Executed:
Auckland, New Zealand.
April 10th 2012

Tony Antunovich, M.D.

PART FOUR

Resources

You have the power to change;

the magic of nature is within reach.

*Embrace it and begin now.*_{PH}

NOTES

1. a) World Health Organization. "Stress in the Work Place." (Retrieved: September 20, 2011) http://www.who.int/occupational_health/topics/ stressatwp/en/.

   b) World Health Organization. "Stress in the Work Place." (Retrieved: September 20, 2011) http://www.who.int/occupational_health/publications/ raisingawarenessofstress.pdf.

2. a) Hammen C. "Stress and Depression." *Annual Review of Clinical Psychology* (2005), 1(1) : 293–319.

   b) Baumann N, Turpin JC. "Neurochemistry of Stress: An Overview." *Neurochemical Research* (2010), 35(12) : 1875–79.

   c) Gazzaniga MS, Ivry RB, Mangun GR. *Cognitive Neuroscience: The Biology of the Mind* (3rd ed.). New York: W.W. Norton, 2008.

   d) Vanderwolf CH. "Brain, Behavior and Mind: What Do You Know and What Can We Know?" *Neuroscience and Biobehavioral Review* (1998), 22(2) : 125–42.

   e) Goldstein DS. "Neurotransmitters and Stress." *Applied Psychophysiology and Biofeedback* (1990), 15(3) : 243–71.

   f) Charney DS. "Psychobiological Mechanisms of Resilience and Vulnerability; Implication for Successful Adaptation to Extreme Stress." *American Journal of Psychiatry* (2004), Focus 2:368–91.

   g) Kronhn HW. *Stress and Coping Theories.* Mainz, Germany: Johannes Gutenberg University, 2005.

3. World Health Organisation. "Investing in Mental Health." http://www.who.int/ mental_health/en/investing_in_mnh_final.pdf (Retrieved: July 15, 2011).

4. National Institute of Mental Health, Statistics. http://wwwapps.nimh.nih.gov/ health/statistics/index.shtml (Retrieved: July 15, 2011).

5. World Health Organisation. "Depression." http://www.who.int/mental_health/ management/depression/definition/en/ (Retrieved: July 15, 2011).

6. World Health Organization. "Suicide Prevention (SUPRE)." http://www.who.int/ mental_health/prevention/suicide/suicideprevent/en/ (Retrieved: July 15, 2011).

7. Mental Health America. "Americans Reveal Top Stressors, How They Cope." http://www.mentalhealthamerica.net/index.cfm?objectid=ABD3DC4E-1372-4D20-C8274399C9476E26# (Retrieved: March 4, 2013).

8. http://www.forbes.com/sites/cywakeman/2013/06/20/the-source-of-your-stress/, http://www.uml.edu/Research/Centers/CPH-NEW/stress-at-work/financial-costs.aspx

9. http://www.stress.org/workplace-stress/ , http://www.workhealth.org/Work%20and%20Health%20Class%202009/09_UHW%20Ch%209.pdf , http://www.uml.edu/Research/Centers/CPH-NEW/stress-at-work/financial-costs.aspx , http://www.stress.org/workplace-stress/

10. a) Mulder EJH, Robles de Medina AC, Huozik BRH, Van der Bergh JK, Buitelaar GH, Visser A. "Prenatal Maternal Stress: Effects on Pregnancy and the (Unborn) Child." *Early Human Development:* Department of Perinatology and Gynaecology, University Medical Center, Ultrect, The Netherland Review: June 28, 2008 (ELSEVIER 2002), 70 : 3–14. Early Human Development (2002), 70 : 3–17.

b) Halligan SL, Herbert J, Goodyer J, Murry M. "Exposure to Postnatal Depression Predicts Elevated Cortisol in Adolescent Offspring." *Biological Psychiatry* (2004), 55(4) : 376–81.

c) Kajantee E. "Fetal Origin of Stress-Related Adults Diseases." *Annals of the New York Academy of Science* (2006), 1083(1) : 11–27.

d) Ball TM, Anderson D, Minto J, Halonen M. "Cortisol Circadian Rhythm and Stress-Response in Infants at Risk of Allergic Diseases." *Journal of Clinical Immunology* (2008), 7(2):306–11.

e) Ali I, Salzberg MR, French C, et al. "Electrophysiological Insights into the Enduring Effects of Early Life Stress On The Brain." *Psychopharmacology* (Berl), (2011), 214(1) : 155–73.

f) Olfman S, ed. *No Child Left Different.* Westport, Conn. Praeger Publishers, 2006.

11. Brain and the milky way: The University of Maine "Children and Brain Develpoment: What we know about What We Know About How Children Learn" – Cooperate Extension Publication _ Bulletin # 4356, Children and Brain Development: What we know about how children learn.

12. a) Graham J. "Children and Brain Develpoment: What we know about What We Know About How Children Learn" The University of Maine. 4356 http://umaine.edu/publications/4356e/

b) Srellpflug C. "Brain Structure". http://www.healingpathwaysmedical.com/docs/Brain_Structure.pdf

13. a) *ScienceDaily,* "Breast milk contain more than 700 species of bacteria, Spanish researchers find". January 4, 2013. http://www.sciencedaily.com/releases/2013/01/130104083103.htm

b) Playford RJ, Macdonald CE, Johnson WS. "Colostrum and milk-derived peptide growth factors for the treatment of gastrointestinal disorders1,2,3,4". *Am.J.Clin.Nutr.* (July 2000), 72(1) : 5-14. http://ajcn.nutrition.org/content/72/1/5.long

c) Gottstein M. "Colostrum is vital ingredient to keep newborn lambs alive". *Irish Independent.* March 3, 2009. http://www.independent.ie/business/farming/colostrum-is-vital-ingredient-to-keep-newborn-lambs-alive-26518112.htm

14. a) http://www.sciencedaily.com/articles/c/colostrum.htm

b) Playford RJ, Macdonald CE, Johnson WS (July 2000). "Colostrum and milk-derived peptide growth factors for the treatment of gastrointestinal disorders". *Am. J. Clin. Nutr.* 72 (1): 5–14. PMID 10871554

c) Gottstein, Michael. Colostrum is vital ingredient to keep newborn lambs alive. *Irish Independent.* 3 March 2009.

d) http://ajcn.nutrition.org/content/72/1/5.full

15. Tesister NS. "Chemotherapy –Induced Oral Mucositis." *Medscape.* April, 2013. http://emedicine.medscape.com/article/1079570-overview

16. a) Gelfraud JM, Neimann A, Daniel B, Shin BA, et al. "Risk of Myocardial Infarction in Patients with Psoriasis." *Journal of the American Medical Association* (JAMA)(2006), 296(14):1735–41.

b) Ivancvich JC. "Maternal Stress and Disruption of Immunity in Utero." WAO: *Medical Journal Review,* 2010. http://www.worldallergy.org/journal_reviews/0410.php

c) Jayson S. "Stress Can Make Allergies Worse" *USA Today.* 14 Aug 2008, http://www.usatoday.com/news/health/2008-08-14-allergies-stress_N.htm.

17. Stress and heart disease:

a) Trophy JM, Lynn C. "Chronic Stress and the Heart Disease.": *JAMA: The Journal of the American Medical Association* (2007), 298 (14) : 1722.

b) Sibai AM, Armenian HK. "Long Term Psychological Stress and Heart Disease" *International Journal of Epidemiology* (2000), 29(5) : 948–49.

Stroke and Stress:

a) Senior K. "Stress Increases Risk of Ischemic Stroke," *Nature Review Neurology* (2009), 5(12) : 635.

b) Surtee PG, Wainwright NW, Luben NW, Wareham NJ, Bingham SA, Khaw KT. "Psychological Distress, Major Depression Disorders and Risk of Stroke."

Neurology(2008), 70(10) : 788–94.

Stress and Fetal Exposure:

a) Sliwowska JH, Verma P, Weinburg J, Hellemans KGC. "Prenatal Alcohol Exposure; Fetal Programming and Later Life Vulnerability to Stress, Depression and Anxiety Disorders." *Neuroscience and Behavioral Reviews* (2010), 34(6) : 791–807

b) Mulder EJ, Robles de Medina PG, Huizink AC, Van der Bergh BRH, Buitelaar JK, Visser GHA. "Prenatal Maternal Stress: Effects on Pregnancy and the (unborn) Child." Department of Perinatology and Gynaeoclolgy, University Medical Center, Ultrect, The Netherlands, Review: 28 June 2008 – Early Human Development – ELSEVIER, (2002), 70 : 3–17.

Stress and Ageing:

a) Cohen S, Janick-Devent D, Miller GE. "Psychological Stress and Disease." *Journal of the American Psychology Association of Science* (2004), 101(49) : 17312–15.

b) Spencer RL, Hutchinson KE. "Alcohol, Ageing and the Stress Response." *Alcohol Research and Health: The Journal of the National Institute on Alcohol Abuse and Alcoholism* (1999), 23(4) : 272.

c) Rosch PJ. "Stress and Aging." *Stress Medicine* (1997), 69–73.

Fertility and Pregnancy:

a) Davis EP, Glynn LM, Dunkel-Scetter C, Hobel C, Chicz-Derment A, and Sandman CA. "Prenatal Exposure to Maternal Depression and Cortisol Influences Infant Temperament." *Journal of American Academy of child and adolescent Psychiatry* (2007), 46(6) : 737–46.

b) Berga S, Brundu B, Loucks L, Adler LJ, Cameron JL. "Increased Cortisol in Cerebrospinal Fluid of Women with Functional Hypothalamic Amenorrhea." *Journal of Clinical Endocrinology and Metabolism* (2006), (Impact:6:2), 91(4) : 1561–65.

c) Epstein RH. "A Conversation With Sarah Berger. A Low-Tech Approach to Fertility: Just-Relax." *New York Times,* September 4, 2007. http://www.nytimes.com/2007/09/04/health/04conv.html.

d) World Health Organization. "Mental Health Aspects of Women's Reproductive Health: A Global Review of Literature." http://whqlibdoc.who.int/publications/2009/9789241563567_eng.pdf.

18. Mental Health America. "Americans Reveal Top Stressors, How They Cope." http://www.mentalhealthamerica.net/index.cfm?objectid=ABD3DC4E-1372-4D20-C8274399C9476E26# (Retrieved: March 4, 2013).

19. a) Murry CJL, Lopez AC. "The Global Burden of Disease of Study: Global Mortality Disability and The Controlling Risk Factor." WHO (1996) Report. *Lancet.* May 17, 1997. 349.

b) Cadwell A. "Lifestyle' Diseases the World's Biggest Killer." http://www.abc. net.au/news/2011-04-28/lifestyle-diseases-the-worlds-biggest-killer/2695712.

c) World Health Organization. "Death from Noncommunicable Diseases on the Rise." http://www.unmultimedia.org/radio/english/2011/04/deaths-from-noncommunicable-diseases-on-the-rise-who-report.

d) Alwan Ala Dr. World Radio Switzerland. "Health Matters: Reducing the Risk of Lifestyle' Diseases." http://worldradio.ch/wrs/programmes/health/health-matters-reducing-the-risks-of-lifestyle-dis.shtml?24328.

e) http://www.un.org/apps/news/story.asp?NewsID=38200&Cr=non-communicable&Cr1.

f) United Nations News Service. "Non-communicable Diseases Leading Cause of Death Worldwide." http://www.un.org/apps/news/story. asp?NewsID=38200&Cr=non-communicable&Cr1.

g) Alwan Ala Dr. "Global Status on Noncommunicable diseases 2010: Description of the Global Burden of NCDs, Their Risk Factors and Determinants." Report of the World Health Organization, (2011).

20. Serotonin:

a) Wutrman RT, Wurtman JJ. "Brain Serotonin, Carbohydrates Craving, Obesity and Depression." *Obesity Research* (1995), 4 : 4775–4805.

b) Sirek A, Sirek OV. "Serotonin: A Review." *Canadian Medical Association Journal.* April 25, 1970. 102(8) : 846–49.

c) Irvine HP. *Serotonin,* Chicago: Medical Publisher, Chicago. 1968.

d) King MW. "Serotonin" *The Medical Biochemistry Page,* Indiana University School of Medicine (2009).

Epinepherine;

a) Kemp SF. "A Review of Causes and Mechanisms." *Journal of Allergy and Clinical immunology* (2002), 110 : 341–48.

b) Roozendaal B. "Stress and Memory: Opposing Effect of Glucocorticoids on Memory Consolidation and Memory Retrieval." *Neurobiology of Learning and Memory* (2002), 78(3):578.

Dopamine:

a) Diehl DJ, Gershon S. "The Role of Dopamine in Mood Disorders." *Comprehensive Psychiatry* (1992), 33(2) : 115–20.

b) Goldstein DS. "Neurotransmitters and Stress." *Applied Psychophysiology and*

Biofeedback (1990), 15(3) : 243–71.

Endorphins:

a) Kotler S. "The Playing Field: Runners High Revisited." *Psychology Today* (20, May 2008).

b) Blake G. "Endorphin Deficiency; Signs and Symptoms." *Nutritional Healing.* WA, Australia.

c) Berk L, Tan SA, [beta]- Endorphin and HGH Increase Are Associated with Both Anticipation and Expression of Mirthful Laughter. *The FASEB Journal* (2006), 20 : A382.

Norepinepherine:

a) Gavin GB. "Stress and Brain Noradrenaline." *Neuroscience and Biobehavioral Review* (1985), 9 : 233–43.

b) Morillak DA, Barrera G, Echevrria DJ, et al. "Role of Brain Norepinephrine in the Bio Behavior Response to Stress." *Progress in Neuro psychopharmacology Biological Psychiatry* (2005), 29(8) : 1214–24.

c) Leonard BE. "Stress, Norepinepherine, and Depression." *Journal of Psychiatry and Neuroscience* (2001), 26(6) : S16.

Melatonin:

a) Solberg EE, Holen A, Ekeberg O, "The Effect of Long Term Meditation on Plasma Melatonin and Blood Serotonin." *Medical Science Monitor* (2004), 10(3), 138–51.

b) Srinivasan V, Smith M, Spence W, Lowe AD, et al. "Melotonin in Mood Disorders." *The World Journal of Biological Psychology,* 7(3) : 138–51.

21. a) Shalala DE. *Mental Health Report: A Report of the Surgeon General- Executive Summary.* National Institute of Mental Health (1999).

b)Brundtland Gro H Dr. *The World Health Report 2001: Mental Health, New Understanding, New Hope.* World Health Organization.

22. Abraham Lincoln, arguably America's greatest and most loved president, sadly suffered from bipolar disorder. See http://www.famousbipolarpeople.com/abraham-lincoln.html

23. a) Effrem K. 'Studies on Effectiveness of Early Childhood Programs." http://edlibertywatch.org/2011/03/studies-on-effectiveness-of-early-childhood-programs

b) Olfman S. ed. *No Child Left Different.* Westport, Conn. Prager Publishers, (2006).

24. Achaan-Chah. "A Still Forest Pool: The Insight Meditation of Achaan Chah." Quest Books. January 1, 2004. P 192.

25. a) Newberg AB, Iverson J. "The Neural Basis of the Complex Mental Task of Meditation: Neurotransmitters and Neurochemical Consideration." *Medical*

Hypotheses Journal (2003), 61(2) : 282–91.

b) Dhammajeva UE. *In This Life Itself: Practical Teachings on Insight Meditation,* Mitrigala, Sanga Publishers, Sri Lanka. http://www.inthislifeitself/udaeriyagama.

26. Parker-Pope T. *NewYorkTimes,* "Human Body is Built for Distance." October 26, 2009. http://www.nytimes.com/2009/10/27/health/27well.html.

27. Running USA: *2011 Marathon, Half Marathon and State Report.* http://www.runningusa.org/node/76115.

28. a) Mader E, Bucher B. "Central pattern generators and the control of rhythmic movements." *ScienceDirect,* November27, 2001. 11(23):986-996. http://www.sciencedirect.com/science/article/pii/S0960982201005814

b) Mondal S, Nandi A. et al. "Modeling a Central Pattern Generator to Generate the Biped Locomotion of a Bipedal Robot Using Rayleigh Oscillators" Indian Institute of Information Technology. 2011. 168: 289-300. http://www.academia.edu/1952963/Modeling_a_Central_Pattern_Generator_to_Generate_the_Biped_Locomotion_of_a_Bipedal_Robot_Using_Rayleigh

c) MacKay-Lyons, M. "Central Pattern Generation of Locomotion: A Review of the Evidence." *The Journal of the American Physical Therapy,* January 2002, 82: 169-83. http://physicaltherapyjournal.com/content/82/1/69.full

29. Lambert GW, Reid C, Kaye DM, Jennings GL, Esler MD. "Effect of sunlight and season on serotonin turnover in the brain". *Lancet* (December 7, 2002), 360(I9348), 1840–1842. http://www.thelancet.com/journals/lancet/article/PIIS0140-6736(02)11737-5/abstract

30. a) Lambert GW, Reid C, Kaye DM, Jennings GL, Esler MD. "Effect of sunlight and season on serotonin turnover in the brain". *Lancet* (December 7, 2002), 360 (19348): 1840–1842. http://www.sciencedirect.com/science/article/pii/S0140673602117375

b) Partonen T. "Vitamin D and Serotonin in winter" *Medial Hypothesis* (September 1998), 51(3) :267-268

31. a) *The Lancet,* December 7, 2002 360 (9348) : 1840–42, doi:10.1016/S0140-6736(02)11737-9

b) Lambert drGW, Reid C, Kaye DM, Jennings GL, Esler MD. "Effect of sunlight and season on serotonin turnover in the brain." http://www.thelancet.com/journals/lancet/article/PIIS0140-6736(02)11737-5/abstract

32. a) http://www.sciencedirect.com/science/article/pii/S0140673602117375

b) http://www.sciencedirect.com/science/article/pii/S0306987798900858

c) Partonen T. "Vitamin D and serotonin in winter", Department of Psychiatry, University of Helsinki, Tukholmankatu 8 C, FIN-00290 Helsinki, Finland

33. a) University of Helsinki," Calcitrol." May13, 1997. http://www.medical-

hypotheses.com/article/S0306-9877(98)90085-8/abstract

b) Harvard Medical School "Two keys to strong bones: Calcium and Vitamin D." November 14, 2013. http://www.health.harvard.edu/healthbeat/two-keys-to-strong-bones-calcium-and-vitamin-d

c) http://www.medical-hypotheses.com/article/S0306-9877(98)90085-8/abstract

d) http://www.sciencedirect.com/science/article/pii/S0306987798900858

34. a) Mackay-Lyons M. "Central Pattern Generation of Locomotion: A Review of the Evidence." *Journal of American Physical Therapy Association.* January 2002. 82:69-83. http://ptjournal.apta.org/content/82/1/69

b) Marder E, Bucher D. "Central pattern generators and the control of rhythmic movements." *ScienceDirect.* November 2001.11(23): 986-996. http://www.sciencedirect.com/science/article/pii/S0960982201005814

c) Mondal S. "Modeling a Central Pattern Generator to Generate the Biped Locomotion of a Biped Robot ..." Indian Institute of Information Technology. http://www.academia.edu/1952963/Modeling_a_Central_Pattern_Generator_to_Generate_the_Biped_Locomotion_of_a_Bipedal_Robot_Using_Rayleigh_Oscillators

35. a) Baker D. *The Powers Latent in Man,* New York: Aquarium Press. 1977, and Newburyport, M. A. *Red Wheel,* Weisner Publishers. 1985.

b) Ober C, Sinatra S, Zucker M. *Earthing: The Most Important Health Discovery Ever?* Laguna Beach, Calif; Basic Health Publications, Inc. 2010.

36. Hammond C. Novous Biologicals. "Ghrelin: Targeting the Hunger Hormone to Combat Obesity and Type 2 Diabetes". http://www.novusbio.com/antibody-news/antibodies/ghrelin-targeting-the-hunger-hormone

37. Hammond C, http://www.novusbio.com/antibody-news/antibodies/ghrelin-targeting-the-hunger-hormone

38. a) CBSNEWS, "Sleep More, Eat Less" November 9, 2014. http://www.bsnews.com/news/sleep-more-eat-less/

b) Cauter EV. "Sleep loss boosts appetite, may encourage weight gain" The Univ, Chicago Medicine. December 6, 2004. http://www.uchospitals.edu/news/2004/20041206-sleep.html

39. a) Taubes G. "Sugar Toxic?" *New York Times,* April 3, 2011. http://www.nytimes.com/2011/04/17/magazine/mag-17Sugar-t.html?.

b) Cohen, E. National Geographic, "Sugar ". August 2013. http://ngm.nationalgeographic.com/2013/08/sugar/cohen-text

c) Jabr F. "Current thoughts on mind, life and culture Is Sugar Really Toxic? Sifting through the Evidence." *Scientific American,* July 7, 2013.

40. a) McCann D, Barrett A, Cooper A, et al. "Food additives and hyperactive

behaviour in 3-year-old and 8/9-year-old children in the community: a randomised, double-blinded, placebo-controlled trial." *The Lancet,* November 3, 2007. 370(9598): 1560-1567. http://www.thelancet.com/journals/lancet/article/PIIS0140673607613063/abstract

b) http://ww.nytimes.com/2011/03/30/health/policy/30fda.html?_r=0

41. Esselstyn C, Campbell TC, Stone G. "Forks over knives, The Experiment" June 2011. P 224.

42. Ecobichon DJ, Joy RM. *Pesticides and Neurological Diseases.* (2nd ed.). Fla; BocaRaton, CRC Press. 1994. pp.335–54.

43. Library of Congress Science Reference Services: *Pesticides and Food.* Tracer Bullet: Science, Technology and on Line. http://www.loc.gov/rr/scitech/tracer-bullets/pestfoodtb.html.

44. Esselstyne C, Campbell TC, Stone G. "Forks over knives, The Experiment" June 2011, P 224.

45. a) Trustwell AS. "The A2 case: a critical review." *European Journal of Clinical Nutrition* (2005), 59: 623-631. http://www.nature.com/ejcn/journal/v59/n5/full/1602104a.html

b) Winkworth CL. "Land-use change and emerging public health risks in New Zealand: assessing Giadia risk." *The New Zealand Medical Journal.* September 10, 2010, 123:1332 http://journal.nzma.org.nz/journal/123-1322/4341/

c) Njoku KL, Akinola MO, Oboh BO. "Phytoremediation Of Crude Oil Polluted Soil: Effect Of Cow Dung Augmentation On The Remediation Of Crude Oil Polluted Soil By Glycine Max." *Journal of Applied Sciences Research.* (2012), 8(1): 277-282.

46. a) Woodford KB Prof. Devil in My Milk: *Illness Health and Politics: A1 and A2 Milk.* Nelson, New Zealand: Craig Potton Publishing, 2007.

b) Fiocchi A, et al, World Allergy Organization (WAO) Diagnosis and Rationale for Action Against Cow's Milk Allergy (DRACMA) Guidelines *WAO Journal* (April 2010). htp://www.worldallergy.org/publications/WAO_DRACMA_guideltines.pdf

c) O'Conner A. The Claim: "Milk Makes you Phlegmy." *New York Times,* Health. April 12, 2010. http://www.nytimes.com/2010/04/13/health/13real.html.

47. Nemec K. "How Milk and Dairy Products Will Destroy Your Health and Cause Cancer, Heart Disease, Diabetes, Multiple Sclerosis, Allergies, Osteoporosis, and Infection." http://www.all-creatures.org/health/howmilkanddairy.html

48. a) Jenkins DJA, Kendal CWC, Augustin LSA, Franceschie S, Hamidi M, Marchie A, Jenkins AL, Axelsen M. "Glycemic Index: Overview of Implication of Health and Disease." *American Journal of Clinical Nutrition.* (2002), 76(1) :

2665–735.

b) Barrett JS, Gibson PR. "Development and Validation of a Comprehensive Semi-Quantitative Food Frequency Questionnaire that Include FODMAOS Intake and Glycemic Index." *Journal of American Diet Association.* October 2010. 110(10):1469–76.

c) Gibson PR, Shepard SJ. "Evidence Based Dietary Management of Functional Gastrointestinal Symptoms: The FODMAPS Approach." *Journal of Gastroenterology and Hepatology* (2010), 25 : 252–58.

49. Mateljan G. *The World's Healthiest Foods: The Essential Guide for the Healthiest Way of Eating.* Seattle, WA. World's Healthiest Food Publisher, 2007.

50. *Guyton's Textbook of Medical Physiology* (8th ed.). Philadelphia: Elsevier Saunders, 1991, 274.

51. Batmanghelidj dr F. *Your Body Cries for Water.* United Kingdom. The Therapist Ltd, 1992.

52. Mayo Clinic: "Nutrition and Healthy Eating: How Much Should You Drink Every Day?" http://www.mayoclinic.com/health/water/NU00283. (Retrieved: September 20, 2011).

53. a) Ewaschuk JB, Levinus DA. "Probiotic and Prebiotic in Chronic Inflammatory Bowel Disease," *World Journal of Gastroenterology* (2006), 12(37) : 594–95. "Probiotics and Prebiotics."

b) *International Journal of probiotics and prebiotics.* New Century Health Publishers. http://www.newcenturyhealthpublishers.com/probiotics_and_ prebiotics/

c) Patel S, Goyal A. "The current trends and future perspectives of prebiotics and research: a review."3 Biotech. June 2012, 2(2): 115-125

54. Mayo Clinic Staff. Slide Show: "How the Digestive System Works." http://www.mayoclinic.com/health/digestive-system/DG00021&slide=7. (Retrieved: September 20, 2011).

55. Bourre JM. "Dietary Omaga 3, Fatty Acids and Psychiatry: Mood, Behaviour, Stress, Depression, Dementia, Aging and Nutrition." *Journal of Nutrition, Health and Aging,* (2005), 14(40) : 64.

56. a) Altman N, "The Honey Prescription." University of Waikato, New Zealand: Healing Arts Press, Rochester, VA. 2010.

b) Molan P, University of Waikatato, NewZealand. 1981. http://manukahoney.com/resources/research/index.html.

57. a) Motala C, Lockey R. "Food Allergy." Allergy Diseases Resource Center, World Allergy Organization. http://www.worldallergy.org/public/allergic_ diseases_center/foodallergy. (Retrieved: September 20, 2011).

b) Keicolt-Glaser JK. "Stress, Food, and Inflammation: Psychoneuroimmunology and Nutrition at the Cutting Edge." *Psychosomatic Medical Journal* (2010), 72(4) : 365–69.

58. Sack RL, Auckly D, Auger RR, Carskdon AM, Write KP, Vitello MV, Zhdsnova IV, "Circadian Rhythm Disorders: Part 1, Basic Principles, Shift Work and Jet Lag Disorders." *An American Academy of Sleep Medicine Review; Sleep* (2007), 30(11) : 1460–83.

59. Sack RL, Auckly D, Auger RR, Carskdon AM, Write KP, et al. "Circadian Rhythm disorders: Part 1, Basic Principles, Shift Work and Jet Lag Disorders." *An American Academy of Sleep Medicine; Sleep* (2007), 30(11) : 1460–83.

60. a) Krahn LE. "Circadian Rhythm Disorders." *Primary Care Sleep Medicine: Current Clinical Practice* (2007) : 261–274.
b) Wagner DR. "Circadian Rhythm Sleep Disorders." *Current Treatment Options in Neurology.* 1(4) : 299–307.
c) Arendt J. "Melatonin Rhythm and Sleep." *New England Journal of Medicine* (2002), 343 : 1114–16.

61. a) http://www.ch.ic.ac.uk/local/projects/s_thipayang/intro.html
b) Imperial College "Melatonin Introduction." http://www.ch.ic.ac.uk/local/projects/s_thipayang/intro.html

62. National Sleep Foundation. "Annual Sleep in America Polls. Exploring Connections with Communication Technology Use and Sleep." (March 7, 2011) http://www.sleepfoundation.org/article/press-release/annual-sleep-america-poll-exploring-connections-communications.

63. Morgenthaler T. "How Many Hours of Sleep are Enough for Good Health?" Mayo Clinic Staff. http://www.mayoclinic.com/health/how-many-hours-of-sleep-are-enough/AN01487. (Retrieved: September 19, 2011).

64. Morgenthaler T. "How Many Hours of Sleep are Enough for Good Health?" Mayo Clinic Staff. http://www.mayoclinic.com/health/how-many-hours-of-sleep-are-enough/AN01487. (Retrieved: September 19, 2011).

65. a) The Stanford Center for Sleep Science and Medicine. "Nighttime Sleep Behaviour". http://stanfordhospital.org/clinicsmedServices/clinics/sleep/sleep_disorders/nighttime-sleep-behaviors.html. (Retrieved: September 19, 2011).
b) Max DT. "The Secret of Sleep." *The National Geographic,* May 2010.

66. a) Anthony CW, Anthony WA. *The Art of Napping at Work,* New York: Larson, 1999.
b) Rees D. "The Biology of Naps: Sleep, Biochemistry and Diet Combine." *Psychology @ 101* (2007). http://dianne-rees.suite101.com/the-biology-of-naps-a30225.

67. Krishnamurthi J. *Choiceless Awareness*. Krishnamurthi Publications of America. December 15, 1992. P158.

68. a) McGee M. "Meditation and Psychiatry." *Psychiatry* (2008), 5(1):28–41.
b) Schooler JW, Smallwood J, Christoff K, Handy TC, Reichle ED, Sayette MA. "Meta-Awareness, Perceptual Decoupling and the Wandering Mind." *Trends in Neuroscience; Trends in Cognitive Science.* 15(7), 319–26.

69. Famous People With Bipolar Disorder, http://bipolar.about.com/od/others/

When you reach the end of your rope,
tie a knot and hang on.
Attributed to Thomas Jefferson[69]
& Abraham Lincoln[22]

REFERENCES

Aaronson RA, Spiro HM. "Mercury and the Gut." (Progress Report). *American Journal of Digestive Diseases* 1973; 18(7): 583 – 94. (Step 6)

Ahnert L, Gunner MR, Lamb ME, Barthel M. "Transition to Child Care: Associations with Infant-Mother Attachment, Infant Negative Emotion and Cortisol Elevations." *Child Development* 2004; 75(3): 639 – 50. (Chapter 2)

Al-Muhsen S, Clarke AE, Kagan RS. "Peanut Allergy: An Overview." *Canadian Medical Association Journal* 2003; 168(10): 1279 – 85. (Step 6)

Álvarez-León EE, Román-Viñas B, Serra-Majem L. "Dairy Products and Health: A Review of the Epidemiological Evidence." *British Journal of Nutrition* 2006; 96: S94 – S99. (Step 6)

American Institute of Stress (AIS). "Stress, Definition of Stress, Stressor, What is Stress?, Eustress?" available at http://www.stress.org/topic-definition-stress. htm, accessed on March 19, 2012. (Chapter 1 and 2)

Anderson GH. "Diet, Neurotransmitters, and Brain Function." *British Medical Bulletin* 1981; 37(1): 95–100. (Steps 2 and 6)

Anthony C, Anthony B. *The Art of Napping at Work* New York: Larson, 1999. (Step 7)

Arias AJ, Steinberg K, Banga A,Trestman RL. "Systematic Review of Efficacy of Meditation Techniques." *Journal of Alternative and Complementary Medicine* 2006; 12(8): 817 – 32. (Step 4)

Armstrong LE. "Rationale for Renewed Emphasis on Dietary Water Intake." *Nutrition Today* 2010; 45(6): S4 – S6. (Step 6)

Babish W. "Stress Hormone in Research on Cardiovascular Effects of Noise." *Noise & Health* 2003; 5(18): 1-11. (Chapter 2)

Banks S, Dinges DF. "Behavioral and Physiological Consequences of Sleep Restriction." *Journal of Clinical Sleep Medicine* 2007; 3(5): 519 – 28. (Step 7)

Baumann N, Turpin JC. "Neurochemistry of Stress: An Overview." *Neurochemical Research* 2010; 35(12): 1875 – 79. (Chapter 3)

Berger M, Gray JA, Roth BL."The Expanded Biology of Serotonin." *Annual Review of Medicine* 2009; 60: 355 – 66. (Chapter 2)

Blow FC, Serras AM, Barry KL. "Late-Life Depression and Alcoholism." *Current Psychiatric Reports* 2007; 9(1): 14 – 19. (Chapter 2)

Bogdanov S, Jurendic T, Sieber R, Gallmann P. "Honey for Nutrition and Health: A Review." *Journal of the American College of Nutrition* 2008; 27(6): 677 – 89. (Step 6)

Bourre JM. "Effects of Nutrients (in Food) on the Structure and Function of the Nervous System: Update on Dietary Requirements for Brain. Part 1: Micronutrients." *Journal of Nutrition Health and Aging* 2006; 10(5): 377 – 85. (Step 6)

Bragg P. *Apple Cider Vinegar: Miracle Health System.* Santa Barbara, CA.: Bragg Books, 2007:Available at http://www.4shared.com/office/dPPjP22P/Apple_Cider_Vinegar_Miracle_He.html, accessed on March 22, 2012. (Step 6)

Brunton PJ, Russell JA. "Neuroendocrine Control of Maternal Stress Responses and Fetal Programming by Stress in Pregnancy." *Progress in Neuro-Psychopharmacology and Biological Psychiatry* 2011; 35(5): 1178 – 91. (Chapter 2)

Chah A. *Unshakeable Peace.* Boston: Wisdom, 2002. (Step 4)

Chang CY, Ke DS, Chen JY. "Essential Fatty Acids and Human Brain." *Acta Neurologica Taiwanica* 2009; 18(4): 231 – 41. (Step 6)

Cohen JL. "Stress and Mental Health: A Biobehavioral Perspective." *Issues in Mental Health Nursing* 2000; 21(2): 185 – 202. (Step 2)

Cohen S, Janicki-Deverts D, Miller GE.. "Psychological Stress and Disease." *Journal of the American Medical Association (JAMA)* 2007; 298(14): 1685 – 87. (Chapter 2)

Cole D, Cole WR, Gaydos SJ, et al. "Aquaculture: Environmental, Toxicological, and Health Issues." *International Journal of Hygiene and Environmental Health* 2009; 212(4): 369 – 77. (Step 6)

Conner KR. "Clarifying the Relationship Between Alcohol and Depression." *Addiction* 2011; 106(5): 915 – 16. (Chapter 6)

Davis JM, Alderson NL, Welsh RS. "Serotonin and Central Nervous System Fatigue: Nutritional Considerations." *American Journal of Clinical Nutrition* 2000; 72(2Suppl): 573S – 78S. (Chapter 2)

De Zoysa P. "The Practice of Mindfulness-Based Behaviour Therapy in Sri Lanka." *Sri Lanka Journal of Psychiatry* 2010; 1(2): 67 – 69. (Step 8)

Dobson H, Ghuman S, Prabhakar S, Smith R. "A Conceptual Model of the Influence of Stress on Female Reproduction." *Reproduction* 2003; 125(2): 151–63. (Chapter 2)

Epstein R. "Fight the Frazzeled Mind: Proactive Steps to Manage Stress." *Scientific American – Mind* (September 8, 2011). (Chapter 1)

Esselsteyn C, Campbell TC, Stone G. *Forks over knives, The Experiment,* 224p. June 2011 13. P

Ewaschuk JB, Dieleman LA. "Probiotic and Prebiotics in Chronic Inflammatory Bowel Diseases". *World Journal of Gastroenterology* 2006; 12(37): 5941 – 50. (Step 6)

Feng X, Wang L, Yang S, Qin D, Wang J, C. Li, et.al.(November 2012). "Maternal separation produces lasting changes in cortisol and behavior in rhesus monkeys." November 2012, 34: 14312–14317. (Chap.3)

Field T, McCabe TP, Schneiderman N, Field TM, eds. *Stress and Coping.* Hillsdale, NJ: Erlbaum, 1985. (Chapters 1 and 2)

Foster-Powel K, Holt SH, Brand-Miller JC. "International Table of Glycemic Index and Glycemic Load Value *American Journal of Clinical Nutrition* 2002; 76(1): 5 - 56. (Step 6 and appendix)

Franklin Institute, Boston Mass. "The Human Brain: Stress on the Brain." http://www.#.edu/learn/brain/stress.html. (Chapter 1)

Fuentes A, Fernandez-Segovia I, Serra JA, Barat JM. "Comparison of Wild and Cultured Sea Bass (Dicentrachus labrax) Quality." *Food Chemistry* 2010; 119(4): 1514 – 18. (Step 6)

Gazzaniga MS, Ivry RB, Mangun GR. *Cognitive Neuroscience: The Biology of the Mind* 3rd ed. New York: W. W. Norton, 2008. (Chapter 1)

Glavin GB. "Stress and Brain Noradrenaline: A Review." *Neuroscience & Biobehavioral Reviews* 1985; 9(2): 233 – 243. (Chapter 2)

Goldstein DS. "Neurotransmitters and Stress." *Biofeedback and Self-Regulation* 1990; 15(3): 243 – 71. (Chapters 2 and 3)

Gunnar M, Quevedo K. "The Neurobiology of Stress and Development." *Annual Review of Psychology* 2007; 58: 145 – 73. (Chapter 2)

Haas EM, Levin B. *Staying Healthy with Nutrition:The Complete Guide to Diet & Nutritional Medicine.* Berkeley, CA: Celestial Arts, 2006. (Step 6)

Halligan SL, Herbert J, Goodyer IM, Murray L. "Exposure to Postnatal Depression Predicts Elevated Cortisol in Adolescent Offspring." *Biological Psychiatry* 2004; 55(4): 376 – 81. (Chapter 2)

Hammen C. "Stress and Depression." *Annual Review of Clinical Psychology* 2005; 1(1): 293 – 319. (Chapter 1)

Harvard School of Public Health. "The Nutrition Source: Protein.," available at www.hsph.harvard.edu/nutritionsource/what-should-you-eat/protein/index.html, accessed on September 19, 2011. (Step 6, Appendix)

Helzer JE, Robins LN, McEvoy L. "Post Traumatic Stress Disorder in the General Population: Findings of the Epidemiologic Catchment Area Survey." *New England Journal of Medicine* 1987; 317(26): 1630 – 34. (Chapter 2)

Hensrud D. *Mayo Clinic Healthy Weight for Everybody*. Mayo Clinic, 2005. (Steps 5 and 6)

Herbert J. "Fortnightly Review. Stress, the Brain, and Mental Illness." *British Medical Journal* 1997; 315(7): 530-35. (Chapters 1 and 2)

Hollmann W, Struder HK. "Brain, Psyche and Physical Activity." *Orthopade* [German] 2000; 29(11): 948 – 56. (Step 5)

Homes TH, Rahe RH. "The Social Readjustment Rating Scale." *Journal of Psychosomatic Research* 1967; 11(2): 213 – 18.

Impey SG, Moor T. "Nutritive Value of Bread Made from Flour Treated with Chlorine Dioxide." *British Medical Journal* 1961; 2(5251): 555 – 56. (Step 6)

Jenkins DJ, Wolever TM, Taylor RH, et al. "Glycemic Index of Foods: A Physiological Basis for Carbohydrate Exchange." *American Journal of Clinical Nutrition* 1981; 34(3): 362 – 66. (Step 6)

Ježová D, Juránková E, Mosnárová A, Kriška M. "Neuroendocrine Response during Stress with Relation to Gender Differences." *ActaNeurobiologiae Experimentalis* 1996; 56(3): 779 – 85. (Chapter 2)

Kaplan BJ, Crawford SG, Field CJ, Simpson JS. "Vitamins, Minerals, and Mood." *Psychological Bulletin* 2007; 133(5): 747 – 60. (Step 6)

Kemp SF, Lockey RF. "Anaphylaxis: A Review of Causes and Mechanisms." *Journal of Allergy and Clinical Immunology* 2002; 110(3): 341 – 48. (Chapter 2)

King DS. "Psychological and Behavioral Effects of Food and Chemical Exposure in Sensitive Individuals." *Nutrition and Health* 1984; 3(3): 137 – 51. (Step 6)

King MW. "Medical Biochemistry Pages on Serotonin Food." Indiana University. Michialking.ph.d/IUschool of Medicine/miking@iupui.edu/1996–2001/ serotonin food. accessed on September 19, 2011.. (Chapters 2 and Step 6)

Knechtle B. "Influence of Physical Activity on Mental Well-Being and Psychiatric Disorders." (German) *Schweitzerische Rundschau fur Medizin Praxis* 2004; 93(35): 1403 – 11. (Step 5)

Kumari M, Head J, Bartley M, Stansfeld S, Kivimaki M. "Maternal separation in childhood and diurnal cortisol patterns in mid-life: findings from the Whitehall II study." July 2012. Psychological Medicine: 633 -37. (Chap.3)

Lakhan SE, Vieira KF. "Nutritional Therapies for Mental Disorders." *Nutrition Journal* 2008; 7(2): unpaginated.. (Step 6)

Lazarus RS, DeLongis A. "Psychological Stress and Coping in Aging." *American Psychologist* 1983; 38(3): 245 – 54. (Chapter 2)

Lechin F, Pardey-Maldonado B, Van der Dijs B, et al. "Circulating Neurotransmitters during the Different Wake-Sleep Stages in Normal Subjects." *Psychoneuroendocrinology* 2004; 29(5): 669 – 85. (Step 7)

Leonard BE. "Stress, Norepinephrine, and Depression." *Journal of Psychiatry & Neuroscience* 2001: 26 Suppl Issue 6 : S16. (Chapter 2)

Lupien SJ, McEwen BS, Gunner MR, Heim C. "Effects of Stress throughout the Lifespan on the Brain: Behavior and Cognition." *Nature Review of Neuroscience* 2009; 10(6): 434 – 45. (Chapter 2)

Ma Q. "Beneficial Effects of Moderate Voluntary Physical Exercise and Its Biological Mechanisms on Brain Health." *Neuroscience Bulletin* 2008; 24(4): 265 – 70. (Step 5)

Mahowald MW, Schenck CH. "Insight from Studying Human Sleep Disorders." *Nature* 2005; 437(7063): 1279 – 85. (Step 7)

Mateljan G. *The World's Healthiest Foods: Essential Guide for the Healthiest Way of Eating.* Seattle, WA: Jessica's Biscuit, 2006. (Step 6)

Mayo Clinic Staff. "Nutrition and Healthy Eating," available at www.mayoclinic. com/health/nutrition-and-healthy-eating/MY00431, accessed on September 19, 2011).

McArdle WD, Katch FI, Katch VL. *Exercise Physiology: Energy, Nutrition, and Human Performance* 4th ed. Baltimore: Williams & Wilkins, 1996. (Steps 5 and 6)

McCarthy S. "Taking Tea: Drink Up (organics: all things purely organic)." *Better Nutrition* 2004; 66(1): 44. (Step 6)

McHugh MP, Cosgrove CH. "To Stretch or Not to Stretch: The Role of Stretching in Injury Prevention and Performance." *Scandinavian Journal of Medicine and Science in Sports* 2010; 20(2):169-181. (Step 5)

McKrell JD. *Treating the Aching Heart: A Guide to Depression, Stress, and Heart Disease.* (book review) *Primary Care Companion to the Journal of Clinical Psychiatry* 2008; 10(6):488 – 89. (Step 2)

Meeusen RK, Watson P, Hasegawa H, Roelands B, Piacenti MF. "Brain Neurotransmitters in Fatigue and Overtraining." *Applied Physiology, Nutrition and Metabolism* 2007; 32(5): 857 – 64. (Step 7)

Meeusen R, de Meirleir K. "Exercise and Brain Neurotransmission." *Sports Medicine* 1995; 20(3): 160 – 88. (Chapter 4 and Step 5)

Mohandas E. "Neurobiology of Spirituality," *Mens Sana Monograph* 2008; 6(1): 63 – 80. (Step 4)

Murray CJ, Lopez AD. "Global Mortality, Disability, and the Contribution of Risk Factors: Global Burden of Disease Study." *Lancet* 1997; 349(9063): 1436 – 42. (Chapter 2)

Mustoe AC, Birnie AK, Korgan AC, Santo JB, French JA (February 2012). "Natural variation in gestational cortisol is associated with patterns of growth in marmoset monkeys (Callithrix geoffroyi)". Gen. Comp. Endocrinol. February 2012. 175 (3): 519–26. (Chap.3)

Institute of Medicine of the National Academies. *Dietary Reference Intakes for Energy, Carbohydrates, Fiber, Fat, Fatty Acids, Cholesterol, Protein, and Amino Acids (Macronutrients)*.Washington, DC; National Academies Press, 2005. (Step 6)

National Digestive Diseases Information Clearinghouse (NDDIC). "How Does Stress Affect IBS?" available at http://digestive.niddk.nih.gov/ddiseases/pubs/ibs/#stress, accessed on March 23, 2012. (Step 6)

Pandit SU. *The State of Mind Called Beautiful.* Boston: Wisdom, 2006. (Step 4)

Pesonen A, Raikkonwn K, Feldtm K, Heinonen K, Osmond C, Philips D, Barker D, Eriksson J, Kajantie E (April 2010). "Childhood separation experience predicts HPA axis hormonal responses in late adulthood: A natural experience of World War II". Psychoneuroendocrinology 35: 785 – 767. (Chap. 3).

Pitt JI. *Fungi and Food Spoilage.* New York: Springer, 2009. (Step 6)

Pollan M. *In Defense of Food: An Eater's Manifesto* London: Penguin, 2009. (Step 6)

Pollock GH. "Chemically Treated Flour." *Journal of the American Medical Association* 1953; 152(11): 1066. (Step 6)

Popkin BM, D'Anci KE, Rosenberg H."Water, Hydration, and Health." *Nutrition Reviews* 2010; 68(8): 439 – 58. (Step 6)

Prasad C. "Food, Mood, and Health: A Neurological Outlook." *Brazilian Journal of Medical and Biological Research* 1998; 31(12): 1517 – 27. (Step 6)

Readers Digest, Editors of. *Fighting Back with Food.* Readers Digest, 2006 (Appendix)

Reading PJ. "Sleep Disorders in Neurology." *Practical Neurology* 2010; 10(5): 300–09. (Step 7)

Rees D. "The Biology of Naps: Sleep, Biochemistry and Diet Combine." http://www.suite101.com/content/the-biology-of-naps-a30225. (Step 7)

Roecklein KA, Rohan KJ. "Seasonal Affective Disorder: An Overview and Update." *Psychiatry (Edgmont)* 2005; 2(1): 20 – 26. (Chapter 2 and Step 5)

Roozendaal B, McEwen BS, Chattarji S. "Stress, Meamory, and the Amygdala." *Nature Review Neuroscience* 2009; 10(6): 423 – 33. (Chapter 2)

Salmon P. "Effects of Physical Exercise on Anxiety, Depression, and Sensitivity to Stress: A Unifying Theory." *Clinical Psychology Review* 2001; 21(1): 33 – 61. (Step 5)

Schmidt MV, Schwab L. "Splintered by Stress: The Good the Bad of Psychological Pressure." Scientific American Mind. August 25, 2011.

Shalala DE. *Mental Health: A Report of the Surgeon General—Executive Summary.* Bethesda, MD, National Institute of Mental Health, 1999, available at http://

www.surgeongeneral.gov/library/mentalhealth/summary.html. accessed on March 28, 2012. (Chapter 2)

Shepard S. *Low Foodmap Diet: Fructose Malabsorption Food Shopping Guide.* Melbourne, Australia: Shepherd Works, 2010. [The webside associated with this book states: "This book is not suitable for use outside of Australia (It is a shopping guide listing Australian foods."] (Step 6)

Shinn SS, Dixon CE. "Oral Fish Oil Restores Striatal Dopamine Release after Traumatic Brain Injury." Neuroscience Letters 2011; 496(3): 168-171.. (Step 6)

Sibai AM, Armenian HK. "Long Term Psychological Stress and Heart Disease." *International Journal of Epidemiology* 2000; 29(5): 948. (Step 2)

Siegel J. "Brain Mechanisms that Control Sleep and Waking." *Naturwissenschaften* 2004; 91(8): 355 – 65. (Step 7)

Silver L, Bassett M. "Food Safety for the 21st Century." *Journal of the American Medical Association* 2008; 300(8): 957 – 59. (Step 6)

Simopoulos AP, ed. *Nutrition and Fitness: Mental Health, Aging, and the Implementation of a Healthy Diet and Physical Activity Lifestyle.* Basel, Switzerland: Karger, 2005. (Steps 5 and 6)

Spencer RL, Hutchinson KE. "Alcohol, Aging and Stress Response." *Alcohol Research and Health* 1999; 23(4): 272 – 283. (Step 2)

Srinivasan V, Smits M, Spence W, et al. "Melatonin in Mood Disorders." *World Journal of Biological Psychiatry* 2006; 7(3): 138 – 51. (Step 7)

Steward O. *Functional Neuroscience.* New York: Springer Verlag, 2000. (Chapter 1)

Suter E, Marti B, Gutzwiller G. "Jogging or Walking: Comparison of Health Effects." *Annals of Epidemiology* 1994; 4(5): 375 – 81. (Step 5)

Takeda E, Terao J, Nakaya Y, et al. "Stress Control and Human Nutrition." *Journal of Medical Investigation* 2004; 51(3-4): 139 – 45. (Step 6)

Tiwari S. "Nature Cure and Yoga". www.naturecureandyoga.com/index.htm. (Retrieved: September 20, 2011). (Step 5 and Appendix)

Torpy JM, Glass RM, Lynm C. "Chronic Stress and the Heart." *JAMA* 2007; 298(14): 1722. (Chapter 2)

Tuormaa TE. "The Adverse Effects of Food Additives on Health: A Review of the Literature with Special Emphasis on Childhood Hyperactivity." *Journal of Orthomolecular Medicine* 1994; 9(4): 225 – 43. (Step 6)

Turcotte M. "Food for Thought: 10 Foods to Increase Your Brain Function." The Diet Channel, available at http://www.thedietchannel.com/Food-For-thought.htm, accessed on October 11, 2006. (Step 6)

Turk FW. "Circadian Rhythms," in Fregly MJ, Blatteis CM. *Handbook of Physiology: Environmental Physiology* 1996 (Step 7)

Walker B. *The Anatomy of Stretching.* Berkeley, CA.: North Atlantic Books, 2007. (Step 5)

Wang J, Korczykowski M, Rao H. et al. "Gender Difference in Neural Response to Psychological Stress." *Social Cognitive and Affective Neuroscience* 2007; 2(3): 227 – 39. (Chapter 2)

World Health Organization. *Global Status Report on Noncommunicable Diseases 2010: Description of the Global Burden of NCDs, Their Risk Factors and Determinants.* Geneva, WHO, 2011, available at http://www.who.int/nmh/publications/ncd_report2010/en/, accessed on March 28, 2012. (Chapter 2)

World Health Organization, Department of Mental Health and Substance Abuse. Promoting Mental Health: Concepts, Emerging Evidence, Practice. Victorian Health Promotion Foundation and University of Melbourne, Geneva, WHO, 2004, available at http://www.who.int/mental_health/evidence/en/promoting_mhh.pdf, accessed on March 28, 2012. HS Saxena, R Moodie (eds.). 2005. (Chapter 2)

World Health Organization. "Global Strategy on Diet, Physical Activity, and Health," Available at http://www.who.int/dietphysicalactivity/strategy/eb11344/strategy_english_web.pdf, accessed on March 28, 2012. (Chapter 2)

Wurtman RJ, Fernstrom JD. "Effects of the Diet on Brain Neurotransmitters." *Nutrition Reviews* 1974; 32(7): 193 – 200. (Step 6)

Young SN. "How to Increase the Serotonin in the Human Brain without Drugs." *Psychiatry and Neuroscience* 2007; 32(6): 394 – 99. (Chapter 2)

GLOSSARY

Acid-Alkaline Balance[1-4]

The balance between acids and bases exerts "a major impact on biochemical reactions and on a variety of physiological processes that are critical for the homeostasis of the entire body and individual cells," writes Walter F Boron in the textbook *Medical Physiology*. Among the amazing qualities of the human body is that the acid-base balance appropriately maintained is different for different cells (in other words, different cells have differences in their resting pH). It is the role of the kidneys and lungs to maintain a healthy balance between acids and bases in the body's fluids.

Acidosis is a condition in which these fluids hold excessive acid. It results either from a buildup of acids or a loss of a bicarbonate (a base), or a combination of these. Healthy lungs help prevent acidosis through the adequate removal of carbon dioxide, an acid: as we breathe out our body is removing excess acids. The kidneys also remove excess acid from the body.

In this book we are concerned primarily with fine-tuning the acid-base balance. Nevertheless, we can learn a great deal about acidosis by looking at disease states associated with more extreme states of acidosis, states in which symptoms are prominent. Thus, recent research suggests that panic attacks, or some panic attacks, may reflect a response by chemosensitive nerve cells attuned to respiration and arousal within the context of acute brain acidosis: Research has shown that carbon dioxide inhalation is capable of provoking panic attacks in some people and carbon dioxide is an acid. Another relevant line of research finds elevated D-lactic acidosis levels in people with chronic fatigue syndrome. Cumulatively these findings suggest acidosis may have an impact on the functioning of the nervous system.

Alkalosis is the opposite condition, in that it occurs when there is too much base in the body fluids. Alkalosis is far less common than acidosis.

Adrenaline
See epinephrine.

Aloe Vera[5-7]
Used medicinally in ancient Egypt, aloe is a common household plant in many parts of the globe. It looks like a cacti, but is softer and more flexible.

Aloe vera -- the best known species of aloe -- produces two substances used for medicinal purposes, gel and latex. The gel is a clear, jelly-like substance found in the inner part of the aloe plant leaf. The latex, which is yellow in color, originates just under the plant's skin. Aloe products formulated from the whole crushed leaf contain both gel and latex. Aloe medications can be taken by mouth or applied to the skin.

According to the U.S. National Library of Medicine, aloe gel is sometimes taken by mouth for osteoarthritis, bowel diseases (including ulcerative colitis), fever, itching, and inflammation, and as a general tonic. In addition, it has been used for stomach ulcers, diabetes, asthma, and as a treatment for some side effects of radiation treatment.

More frequently, the gel is used topically for such skin conditions as burns, sunburn, frostbite, psoriasis, and cold sores, as well as for the healing of surgical wounds and bedsores.

Aloe latex taken my mouth is considered likely unsafe, especially at high doses, according to the US National Library of Medicine. Whole-leaf aloe may be carcinogenic.

There are preliminary studies in laboratory animals suggesting that some of the chemicals found in aloes may have beneficial effects on the immune system. It is important in Oxidative Stress relief.

The US National Center for Complementary and Alternative Medicine and the US National Library of Medicine at the National Institutes of Health caution that people with diabetes who use glucose-lowering medication should be cautious about oral aloe as it may affect blood glucose levels. Further, all types of oral aloe products may be unsafe for children and for pregnant or breast-feeding women, although the evidence is not definitive. There are reports of people who have taken aloes orally for a few weeks or longer who have developed hepatitis. Aloe injections may be implicated in some way in the deaths of several people.

Side effects of oral aloe may include abdominal pain, nausea and vomiting, diarrhea, and electrolyte (chemical) imbalance in the blood; the use of high doses of aloes appears to increase the likelihood that such side effects may occur.

Much remains to be learned about aloe vera and there may be great benefit hidden here, but at present excessive use is not guaranteed to be benign.

Cortiosol[8-12]

Sitting on top of the kidneys, the adrenal glands secrete many hormones, cortisol being among them. Cortisol is beneficial in that it helps the human body use sugar and protein for energy, and in this way empowers our bodies to recover from infections, surgical procedures, and physical and emotional stress.

However, when stress is prolonged, excessive cortisol secretion may occur. This may lead to a condition of sustained and chronic elevation of cortisol levels, with harmful consequences. For example, exposing the human brain to elevated cortisol levels over extended periods of time may adversely affect the connections between nerve cells. For another example, the prolonged, stress-induced secretion of cortisol may lead to abdominal obesity and metabolic changes that increase insulin secretion as well as levels of harmful blood lipids.

Relaxation techniques and other helpful approaches to stress management benefit us by reducing cortisol levels, while at the same time lowering blood pressure levels, strengthening the immune system, and alleviating anxiety and depression.

Dopamine[13-17]

Dopamine levels in the brain strongly affect our feelings of pleasure, reward, and reinforcement, while also playing an important role in movement (and the coordination of body motion), attention, and memory. Dopamine exerts wide-ranging effects, having important homeostatic functions and being active in establishing global brain states. Several different parts of the brain are particularly sensitive to the effects of dopamine, including the midbrain, the cerebral cortex, and the hypothalamus.

Natural, healthy living with adequate sleep creates dopamine levels without harmful effects. However, understanding how drugs that cause damage to the human body create positive feelings and cause addiction can help us grasp the power of dopamine. The effect of elevated dopamine levels is illustrated by how attractive cigarette smoking has proven to be, as nicotine causes the release of dopamine in the brain. Drugs such as cocaine, methamphetamine, and amphetamine also affect dopamine levels, while causing great damage to the body.

An extreme example of the effects of low dopamine levels appears in Parkinson's disease, an illness characterized by the death or damaging of dopamine-producing brain cells.

Endorphins[18-21]

The US Centers for Disease Control and Prevention describes endorphins as "the natural 'feel-good' chemicals in the body, because they leave you with a naturally happy feeling." Endorphins are active in such natural activities as eating, drinking, exercise, sports, sex, and maternal activities.

Endorphins are created primarily in the pituitary gland in the brain. Recent research suggests that certain cells of the immune system also produce endorphins. They exert their pain-reducing effects primarily at mu-subtype opioid receptors, which are located not only in the central nervous system but also throughout the peripheral nervous system. That endorphins and norepinephrine function in the gastrointestinal tract is related to why in stressful situations a person, may feel 'a tightening in the stomach' while when tension is released the gut relaxes. In the central nervous system they participate in a cascade of chemical reactions that leads to increased production of dopamine, a hormone associated with pleasure.

Understanding how endorphins were discovered, a few decades ago may help us understand what they are and what they do. Scientists asked themselves the following question: Why did the nerves of the human body evolve to have a way of receiving the chemicals in opium and using those chemicals to generate feelings? That question led scientists to the discovery of the specific binding sites in the brain occupied by opiates. The next question posed was why would there be opium receptors unless there were natural substances produced by the human body that would have morphine-like properties? These substances with their pain-relieving properties are what we now call "endorphins."

Epinephrine/Adrenaline[22-25]

Epinephrine, also known as adrenaline, is released by the body in stressful situations. For example, if you were going to take a test or walk up to the plate to bat while playing baseball, your adrenal glands would release epinephrine. It would speed your heart rate, which would increase the amount of oxygen available to your muscles, permitting your body to react faster and better; it would act on your lungs to enable increased ventilation; it would act in the liver to maintain the supply of glucose in the blood needed for your muscles to contract and for your brain to direct your activities; and would decrease insulin levels, which would also help to maintain blood sugar levels.

Furthermore, epinephrine appears to play a role in the secretion within the brain of the hormones oxytocin and vasopressin. Vasopressin has numerous functions, ranging from stimulating the contraction of capillaries and arterioles to raise blood pressure, to promoting contraction of parts of the intestines, to helping to contract the uterus, to affecting the collecting tubules of the kidneys. Oxyctocin functions during labor and the expression of milk.

While epinephrine, norepinephrine, and serotonin are all neurotransmitters, epinephrine functions at a lower level in the brain than the others and acts upon fewer of the nerve cells of the brain.

A relatively limited number of nerve cells in the medulla of the brain convert norepinephrine into epinephrine.

Genetically Modified (GM) Products[26-27]

Genetic modification involves the application of a specialized toolbox using recent technologies to alter the genetic makeup of animals, plants, or bacteria. (Other phrases used to describe such products are "genetically engineered" or "transgenic.") A genetically modified product contains genes from SEVERAL different organisms. At present, genetic modification has been applied to create new medicines and vaccines, foods and food ingredients, feeds, and fibers. In 2006, 252 million acres of transgenic crops were planted in 22 countries by 10.3 million farmers. Among the crops most likely to be genetically modified are soybeans, corn, cotton, canola, and alfalfa.

Most GM crops possess advantages not found in conventional plants: in particular, herbicide resistance and insect resistance. But while some of the advantages of genetically modified crops are readily seen, there may be unknown or unforeseen risks. A swirl of controversy surrounds GM foods, and it seems unlikely that all the important questions will find speedy resolution.

Hormones[28-30]

The human body's chemical messengers, hormones are produced in the glands and sent out through the bloodstream. Hormones function as an array of regulatory molecules that transmit specific information among cells and among organs. Such molecular communication takes place in humans with a considerable level of complexity, with hormones, neurotransmitters, immune-system components and other parts of us all interacting.

Some hormones regulate the immune system. Some act within neurons, where they function as neurotransmitters. No surprise then that hormones affect numerous processes and illnesses. For example, as is fairly well known, hormonal changes appear to influence both the triggering and frequency of migraine headache attacks in women.

"Hormones are powerful," the US National Library of Medicine at the National Institutes of Health explains. Even small amounts of a hormone are capable of generating large changes in the cells of the body, or even in the entire body.

Lavender[31-33]

Yes, the beautiful lavender plant is an herb. And both the lavender flower and the oil of lavender are used in formulating medicines.

According to the US National Library of Medicine, lavender

is used for restlessness, insomnia, anxiety, nervousness, and depression. In addition, there are a number of digestive illnesses for which people look to lavender: for example abdominal swelling from gas, loss of appetite, vomiting, nausea, intestinal gas (flatulence), and upset stomach.

Among the additional uses for which some people find lavender helpful are migraine headaches, toothaches, sprains, nerve pain, sores, joint pain and acne. Some use it to promote menstruation. Some use it during cancer therapy.

Lavender may be applied to the skin and is sometimes used for hair loss (alopecia areata) and pain, as well as to repel mosquitoes and other insects. Lavender may be added to bathwater and some people are doing so to treat circulation disorders and to improve mental well being. Aromatherapy with lavender is used for insomnia, pain, and agitation related to dementia.

Lavender oil has sedating effects and may encourage muscle relaxation, the National Library of Medicine explains. Using lavender oil in a vaporizer overnight may benefit people with mild insomnia. Similarly, bathing in water to which 3 mL of a mixture of 20 percent lavender oil and 80 percent grapeseed oil has been added may benefit mood.

Notably, related plant species are sometimes permitted to contaminate pure lavender.

The US National Library of Medicine points to studies suggesting effectiveness for lavender but also points to potential side effects. "Lavender is likely safe for most adults in food amounts and possibly safe in medicinal amounts." Known side effects of oral lavender include constipation, headache, and increased appetite. Lavender oil products applied to the skin have been known to cause abnormal breast growth in young boys.

In adults, the power of lavender to slow down the central nervous system may be a factor relevant to surgical procedures: Lavender may cause harm if used in combination with anesthesia and other medications administered during surgery. Thus, lavender use should be stopped at least 2 weeks prior to scheduled surgery. Another caution is that lavender should not be used with the following medications, as adverse effects may result: barbiturates, chloral hydrate, and such sedatives as clonazepam (Klonopin), lorazepam (Ativan), phenobarbital (Donnatal), zolpidem (Ambien), and others.

Melatonin[34-37]

Melatonin, a hormone that promotes normal sleep, is produced by the pineal gland in the human brain, the production being synchronized with the light-dark cycle. A considerable body of research on melatonin as a sleep aid has shown that its impact on insomnia is real but relatively small. Studies with elderly persons suffering from insomnia indicate that melatonin can help them fall asleep faster; for younger people with insomnia there may also be benefit, although this is not as certain.

For those whose sleep problems involve an inability to sleep during the nighttime, that is, people with what is known as a circadian rhythm abnormality, melatonin shows greater effectiveness. Such people might take 3 mg of melatonin 4 to 5 hours before the time they wish to start sleeping.

Other groups of people who may benefit from melatonin therapy are those with jet lag and those engaged in shift work. Thus, for example, people who travel across five or more time zones, and particularly people who so travel in an eastward direction, may benefit from melatonin (3 mg at 4 to 5 hours prior to the time they wish to start sleep).

The safety of melatonin for short-term use seems relatively certain. However, there are two types of melatonin available: natural and synthetic (man-made). As the natural melatonin derives from the glands of animals and can be contaminated with a virus, the American Academy of Family Physicians recommends the synthetic form. Also, while melatonin is relatively safe there have been reports of excess sleepiness, headache, stomach discomfort, depression, a "hung-over" feeling, and a "heavy-head" feeling.

Dietary supplements with melatonin "precursors," L-tryptohhan and 5-HTP, appear not to be safe. Nor have they proven effective for insomnia. [L-tryptophan is an amino acid that the body converts to 5-HTP, and this, in turn, is converted to serotonin and then to melatonin.) Furthermore, they appear not to be safe. Both of these products may be linked to a complex debilitating systemic condition known as eosinophilia-myalgia syndrome (EMS).

Neurochemicals[38]

A nerve cell has a central cell body and various arms that perform a variety of functions. The cell body contains an extremely sophisticated biosynthesis apparatus that forms enzymes and other chemicals necessary for the proper functioning of the nerve. As nerves activate, the substances produced by the biosynthesis apparatus serve to replenish those molecules and other substances secreted by the nerve cell and those inactivated during neural activity.

Thus it is important to understand that the numerous neurotransmitters active in the nerves are no more than a portion of the substances that must work together for the healthy functioning of the nerves.

Neurotransmitters[39-41]

Nerve cells communicate with one another across a tiny space called a synapse: that is where signals move from one nerve cell to another. The chemical messengers released at the synapse to permit communication between nerve cells are called neurotransmitters. There are more than fifty neurotransmitters, and perhaps many more than that.

Thus, a minute sac of chemicals at the end of one arm of a nerve releases neurotransmitters into the space (the synapse) between two nerve cells and these chemicals – the neurotransmitters -- cross the synapse and attach to receptors on the neighboring cell, changing properties in this cell.

Some neurotransmitters make other cells more excitable; these neurotransmitters help make muscles contract and glands secrete hormones. Other neurotransmitters exert an inhibitory effect, making cells less excitable; these neurotransmitters help to control muscle activity while also playing an important role in the human visual system.

An important example of what neurotransmitters do is how they help control sleep and wakefulness, which they accomplish by acting on groups of nerve cells. Serotonin and norepinephrine are among the neurotransmitters that ensure that certain parts of the brain are active when we are awake.

Norepinephrine[42-45]

Norepinephrine is a neurotransmitter that plays a key role in communication among brain cells. Notably, norepinephrine exerts both excitatory and inhibitory effects on various portions of the central nervous system as well as on more peripheral nerve cells, with effects on such factors as the firing rates of nerve cells.

Norepinephrine functions prominently in the sleep-wake cycle; affects sensory processing, movement, mood, memory, and anxiety; and has a key role in regulating blood volume and blood pressure. The midbrain, cerebral cortex, and hypothalamus are among the parts of the brain that are particularly sensitive to norepinephrine levels.

Low levels of norepinephrine may be associated with depressed mood. It is revealing that the effect of many antidepressant medications is to increase levels of norepinephrine and/or serotonin and other neurotransmitters in the brain. These same medications that affect noreipnephrine and serotonin levels are used to treat anxiety disorders. That cocaine, methamphetamine, and amphetamine affect norepinephrine levels illustrates some of the power norepinephrine and these other neurotansmitters possess.

A major illness that is characterized by inadequate norepinephrine levels is Parkinson's disease, where the nerve endings responsible for producing norepinephrine suffer impairment.

Oxidative Stress[46-49]

Physiological stress on the body that is caused by the cumulative damage done by free radicals inadequately neutralized by antioxidants and that is held to be associated with aging.[46] It reflects an imbalance between the systemic development of reactive oxygen, and the biological system's ability to readily detoxify the reactive intermediates, or to repair the resulting damage on a cellular level.

Reactive oxygen species (ROS) are highly reactive molecules that consist of a number of diverse chemical species including superoxide anion ($O2-$), hydroxyl radical ($-OH$), and hydrogen peroxide ($H2O2$). Because of their potential to cause oxidative deterioration of DNA, protein, and lipid, ROS have been implicated as one of the causative factors of aging.[47]

As ROS are generated mainly as by-products of mitochondrial

respiration, mitochondria are thought to be the primary target of oxidative damage and play an important role in aging. Emerging evidence has linked mitochondrial dysfunction to a variety of age-related diseases, including neurodegenerative diseases and cancer.[48]

Oxidative stress attacks mitochondria, leading to increased oxidative damage. As a consequence, damaged mitochondria progressively become less efficient, losing their functional integrity and releasing more oxygen molecules, increasing oxidative damage to the mitochondria, and culminating in an accumulation of dysfunctional mitochondria with age.[49]

Phytoremediation[50-54]

Phytoremediation is defined as the use of green plants to remove pollutants from the environment or to render them harmless or a process of decontaminating soil or water by using plants and trees to absorb or break down pollutants.[50]

Around the world, there is an increasing trend in areas of land, where surface waters and groundwater is affected by contamination from industrial, military and agricultural activities either due to ignorance, lack of vision, or carelessness.

Harvesting plants on a contaminated site as a remediation method is a passive technique that can be used to clean up sites with shallow, low to moderate levels of contamination. Phytoremediation can be used to clean up metals, pesticides, solvents, explosives, crude oil, polyaromatic hydrocarbons, and landfill leachates. It can also be used for river basin management through the hydraulic control of contaminants.[51]

The uptake of contaminants in plants occurs primarily through the root system. Plant roots also cause changes at the soil-root interface as they release inorganic and organic compounds (root exudates) in the rhizosphere. These root affect a number of activities of the microorganisms, and the aggregation and stability of the soil.

Often toxic substances enter the food chain via grazers, such as cows and other livestock, that feed on plants grown in contaminated soils. The toxins then accumulated and concentrated in the meat and milk products eventually consumed by humans.[52]

An example being, Selenium(Se) contamination of soil. The irrigation and drainage of water is one of the most serious problems confronting the western United States and other parts of the world. It damages birds and wild life and is detrimental to all.

Researchers are developing three types of Indian mustard (Brassica Juncea), to remove Se and heavy metals from the soil. Cd and Zn were some of the other heavy metals extracted from the soil. The Mustard plant is able to absorb 25% of more metal than other plants.[53] We need to have awareness we do not consume these plants, which would accumulate in our bodily system.

Serotonin[55-62]

Serotonin is an inhibitory neurotransmitter. According the US National Institute of Neurological Disorders and Stroke, it is **present throughout the body and brain; seven subtypes of serotonin receptors have been identified in the brain. Serotonin strongly affects the functioning of the midbrain, cerebral cortex, and hypothalamus.**

Serotonin levels influence our mood, sexual desire, and appetite. It has a role in constricting blood vessels, lowering the pain threshold, and in regulating both body temperature and sleep. It plays an important role in headache, vomiting, alcoholism, and pain disorders Deficiency of serotonin underlies depression and other mood and behavior disorders, as well as associated sleep disorders. It is notable that serotonin functions as a precursor for the synthesis of melatonin by the body.

Knowing that several antidepressant drugs influence levels of serotonin, norepinephrine, and dopamine tells us something about what serotonin's effect on us. And when doctors prescribe antidepressants for people with obsessive-compulsive disorder, the only medicines found to work well are those that affect serotonin levels. The power of serotonin is illustrated by the fact that such harmful drugs as cocaine, LSD, and ecstasy (MDMA) alter serotonin levels, as do medicines used to treat acute episodes of migraine headache.

Stress[63-65]

"For some time it has been clear that psychosocial states such as stress, social isolation, and depression alter the risk of developing chronic illness and increase the risk of adverse outcomes," writes Mary Charlson in a leading standard textbook of medicine. A large body of medical research has demonstrated the impact of chronic stress on the structure and function of the brain, particularly upon those parts of the brain called the hippocampus, amygdale, and prefrontal cortex. Important in threat recognition, in fear, and in emotional learning, the amygdala and prefrontal cortex are associated with the affective and attentional responses to stress.

Thus, for example, chronic stress may interfere with problem solving. And as the hippocampus serves several types of memory, severe stress may affect memory and impede a person's ability to evaluate the seriousness of a potential threat. And while stress can actually reduce the size of the hippocampus, there is evidence that exercise and enriched environments have the potential to lead to the appearance of new cells. Recent research has demonstrated that chronic stress has a negative impact upon telomere length (Telomeres being specialized DNA sequences that serve as tiny caps located at the end of chromosomes).

It is important to remember that stressful events occur in the life of every person and that how each of us views those events and how we address them and how we seek social support influences their impact on us. None of us responds to stressful events outside the context of how our society and, more specifically, how our own social network views such events.

Reducing levels of stress is a healthy approach to many of life's problems. As this book shows, people can learn how to better handle stress.

Tea Tree Oil[66-68]

Centuries ago, sailors who made tea from the leaves of a tree on the southeast coast of Australia named the tree the "tea tree."It is oil derived from those leaves that is now called tea tree oil.

Tea tree oil is applied to the skin as a treatment for acne and other infections, and is used for infections of the nail (onychomycsis), for lice, scabies, athlete's foot (tinea pedis) and ringworm; for cuts and abrasions, burns, insect bites and stings, and boils. It is also used for vaginal infections, recurrent herpes labialis, toothache, infections of the mouth and nose, sore throat, otitis media, otitis externa, and other ear infections. Some people add tea tree oil to bath water to treat cough, bronchial congestion, and pulmonary inflammation.

According to the US National Library of Medicine there is some scientific evidence that application of a sufficiently strong preparation carries some effectiveness for athlete's foot (tinea pedis), for fungus infections of the nails, and for acne.

Applying tea tree oil preparations to the skin is likely safe for most people, according to the US National Library of Medicine, although there have been reports of skin irritation and swelling. Used for acne, it may cause skin dryness, itching, stinging, burning, and redness.

TEA TREE OIL SHOULD NOT BE TAKEN BY MOUTH. There are reports of oral use leading to confusion, inability to walk, unsteadiness, drowsiness, confusion, hallucinations vomiting, diarrhea, stomach upset, blood cell abnormalities, weakness, rash, and coma. When ingested, tea tree oil can be toxic.

Trans Fats[69-71]

Certain foods contain trans fat, a type of cooking fat that, through a process called hydrogenation, combines hydrogen with vegetable oil. Trans fats increase the shelf life of foods and make foods taste less greasy. Foods more likely to contain trans fats are chips, crackers, cookies, muffins, sweet rolls, deep-fried food purchased commercially, microwave popcorn, shortenings, and stick margarine.

Trans fats have an unhealthy impact on the fats circulating through your blood. In addition, there is some evidence that trans fats may damage the cells lining blood vessels and may increase inflammation; and both of these processes may lead to blockages of the blood vessels of the heart. Because of the harmful and potentially harmful effects of trans fats, the US Food and Drug Administration now requires food manufacturers to list trans fat on the Nutrition Facts panels appearing on many foods.

Glossary References

1. US National library of Medicine, "Acidosis," available at http://www.nlm.nih.gov/medlineplus/ency/article/001181.htm, accessed on March 26, 2012.
2. Wemmie JA. "Neurobiology of Panic and pH Chemosensation in the Brain," *Dialogues in Clinical NeuroSciences* 2011; 13(4): 475-83.
3. Sheedy JR, Wettenhall RE, Scanlon D, et al. "Increased Lactic Acid Intestinal Bacteria in Patients with Chronic Fatigue Syndrome." *In Vivo* 2009; 23(4): 621-28.
4. Boron WF. "Acid-Base Physiology," in Boron WF, Bowlpaep EL. *Medical Physiology* 2nd ed. Philadelphia, Saunders, 2009.
5. US National Library of Medicine, "Aloe" available at http://www.nlm.nih.gov/

medlineplus/druginfo/natural/607.html, accessed on March 20, 2012.

6. National Center for Complementary and Alternative Medicine, "Aloe Vera," available at http://nccam.nih.gov/health/aloevera, accessed on March 20, 2012.

7. American Cancer society, "Aloe," available at http://www.cancer.org/Treatment/TreatmentsandSideEffects/ComplementaryandAlternativeMedicine/HerbsVitaminsandMinerals/index, accessed on March 22, 2012.

8. Clinical Center, National Institutes of Health, "Managing Adrenal Insufficiency."Available at http://www.nlm.nih.gov/medlineplus/ency/article/003693.htm, accessed on March 20, 2012.

9. National Institutes of Health Clinical Center, "Managing Adrenal Insufficiency," accessed at http://www.cc.nih.gov/ccc/patient_education/pepubs/mngadrins.pdf. on March 20, 2012.

10. Linker E. "Insulin Resistance and the Metabolic Syndrome," in Rakel D. *Integrative Medicine* 2nd ed. Philadelphia, Saunders, 2007.

11. Cullum-Dugan D, Saper RB. "Obesity," in Rakel D. *Integrative Medicine* 2nd ed. Philadelphia, Saunders, 2007.

12. Kligman EW. Maintaining Health and Aging Optimally," in Rakel D. *Integrative Medicine* 2nd ed. Philadelphia, Saunders, 2007.

13. Purves D, Augustune GJ, Fitzpatrick D, et al. *Neuroscience* 4th ed. Sunderland, MA; Sinauer Associates, 2008.

14. Robinson K, Lang EJ, "The Nervous System," in Koeppen BM, Stanton BA. *Berne & Levy Physiology* 6th ed. Philadelphia, Mosby, 2008.

15. The Mayo Clinic. "Parkinson's disease," available at http://www.mayoclinic.com/health/parkinsons-disease/DS00295/DSECTION=causes, accessed on March 26, 2012.

16. The Mayo Clinic: "Nicotine Dependence: Causes," available at http://www.mayoclinic.com/health/nicotine-dependence/DS00307/DSECTION=causes, accessed on March 26, 2012.

17. US National Institutes of Health. National Institute on Drug Abuse. "Impact of Drugs on Neurotransmission," available at http://www.drugabuse.gov/news-events/nida-notes/2007/10/impacts-drugs-neurotransmission accessed on March 26, 2012.

18. US Centers for Disease Control and Prevention. "Feelin Frazzled...?," available at http://www.bam.gov/sub_yourlife/yourlife_feelingfrazzled.html, accessed on March 26, 2012.

19. Sprouse-Blum AS, Smith G, Sugai D, Parsa FD. "Understanding Endorphins and Their Importance in Pain management," *Hawaii Medical Journal* 2010; 69: 70-71.

20. Mulroney SE, Myers AK. *Netter's Essential Physiology* Philadelphia, Saunders, 2009.

21. National Alliance of Methadone Advocates, "The Discovery of Endorphins," available at http://www.methadone.org/library/woods_1994_endorphin.html, accessed on March 26, 2012.

22. Gengo FM. "Pharmacological Principles in Treating Neurological Disease," in Bradley WG, Daroff RB, Fenichel GM, Janovic J. *Neurology in Clinical Practice* 5th ed. Butterworth-Heinemann, 2008.

23. Purves D, Augustune GJ, Fitzpatrick D, et al. *Neuroscience* 4th ed. Sunderland, MA; Sinauer Associates, 2008.

24. US National Library of Medicine, "Epinephrine and exercise," available at http://www.nlm.nih.gov/medlineplus/ency/anatomyvideos/000051.htm, accessed on March 26, 2012.

25. Barrett E. "The Adrenal gland," in Boron WF, Bowlpaep EL. *Medical Physiology* 2nd ed. Philadelphia, Saunders, 2009.

26. Human Genome Project Information, "Genetically Modified Foods and Organisms," available at http://www.ornl.gov/sci/techresources/Human_Genome/elsi/gmfood.shtml, accessed on March 20, 2012.

27. World Health Organization, "Food Safety: 20 Questions on Genetically Modified Foods," available at http://www.who.int/foodsafety/publications/biotech/20questions/en/, accessed on March 20, 2012.

28. US National Library of Medicine, "Hormones," available at http://www.nlm.nih.gov/medlineplus/hormones.html, accessed on March 20, 2012.

29. National Headache Foundation, "Hormones and Migraine," available at http://www.nlm. nih.gov/medlineplus/hormones.html, accessed on March 20, 2012.

30. Habener JF, "Genetic Control of Peptide Hormone Formation ," in Melmed S, Polonsky KS, Larsen PR, Kronenberg HM. *Williams Textbook of Endocrinology*, 12th ed. Philadelphia, Saunders, 2011.

31. US National Library of Medicine, "Lavender" available at http://www.nlm.nih.gov/medlineplus/druginfo/natural/838.html, accessed on March 22, 2012.

32. US National Institutes of Health, National Center for Complementary and Alternative Medicine, "Lavender," available at http://nccam.nih.gov/health/lavender/ataglance.htm. accessed on March 22, 2012.

33. US Department of Health and Human Services, National Institutes of health, National Center for Complementary and Alternative Medicine. "Herbs at a Glance: A Quick Guide to Herbal Supplements," available at http://nccam.nih.gov/sites/nccam.nih.gov/files/herbs/NIH_Herbs_at_a_Glance.pdf, accessed on March 22, 2012.

34. US National Institutes of Health, National Center for Complementary and Alternative Medicine, "Sleep Disorders and CAM: At a Glance," available at, http://nccam.nih.gov/health/sleep/ataglance.htm, accessed on March 25, 2012.

35. Mahowald MW. "Disorders of Sleep," in Goldman L, Schafer AI, *Cecil Medicine,* 24th ed, Philadelphia, Elsevier, 2011.

36. US National Library of Medicine, "Melatonin," available at http://www.nlm.nih.gov/medlineplus/druginfo/natural/940.html, accessed on March 25, 2012.

37. American Academy of Family Physicians. "Melatonin," available at http://familydoctor.org/familydoctor/en/drugs-procedures-devices/over-the-counter/melatonin.printerview.all.html, accessed on March 26, 2012.

38. Robinson K, Lang EJ, "The Nervous System," in Koeppen BM, Stanton BA. *Berne & Levy Physiology* 6th ed. Philadelphia, Mosby, 2008.

39. Robinson K, Lang EJ, "The Nervous System," in Koeppen BM, Stanton BA. *Berne & Levy Physiology* 6th ed. Philadelphia, Mosby, 2008.

40. US National Institute of Neurological disorders and Stroke, "Brain Basics: Know Your Brain," available at http://www.ninds.nih.gov/disorders/brain_basics/know_your_brain.htm, accessed on March 20, 2012.

41. US National Institute of Neurological Disorders and Stroke, "Brain basics: Understanding Sleep," available at http://www.ninds.nih.gov/disorders/brain_basics/understanding_sleep.htm, accessed on March 20, 2012.

42. Gengo FM. "Pharmacological Principles in Treating Neurological Disease," in Bradley WG, Daroff RB, Fenichel GM, Janovic J. *Neurology in Clinical Practice* 5th ed. Butterworth-Heinemann, 2008.

43. The Mayo Clinic. "Depression (Major Depression): Serotonin and Norepinephrine Reuptake Inhibitors (SNRIs)," available at http://www.mayoclinic.com/health/antidepressants/MH00067. accessed on March 26, 2012.

44. The Mayo Clinic. "Parkinson's disease," available at http://www.mayoclinic.com/health/parkinsons-disease/DS00295/DSECTION=causes, accessed on March 26, 2012.

45. US National Institutes of Health. National Institute on Drug Abuse. "Impact of Drugs on Neurotransmission," available at http://www.drugabuse.gov/news-events/nida-notes/2007/10/impacts-drugs-neurotransmission. accessed on March 26, 2012.

46. http://www.merriamwebster.com/medical/oxidative%20stress

47. Gemma, C. Vila, J. Bachstetter, A. Bickford,P. "Oxidative Stress and Ageing Brain: From Theory to Prevention. NBIC Resources. 2007. Chap 15. http://www.ncbi.nlm.nih.gov/books/NBK3869/

48. Hang, C. Kong, Y. Zhan, H. "Oxidative Stress, Mitochondrial Dysfunction, and Aging." J. Signal Transduct. October 2,2012 : 646354. http://www.ncbi.nlm.nih.gov/pmc/articles/PMC3184498/

49. Hang, C. Kong, Y. Zhan, H. "Oxidative Stress, Mitochondrial Dysfunction, and Aging." J. Signal Transduct. October 2,2012 : 646354. http://www.ncbi.nlm.nih.gov/pmc/articles/PMC3184498/

50. http://dictionary.reference.com/browse/phytoremediation
51. http://www.unep.or.jp/Ietc/Publications/Freshwater/FMS2/1.asp
52. http://www.mhhe.com/biosci/pae/botany/botany_map/articles/article_10.html
    Phytoremediation: Using plants to clean soil, Botany Global Issue Map. February 2000.
53. http://www.mhhe.com/biosci/pae/botany/botany_map/articles/article_10.html
54. http://chemistry.armstrong.edu/nivens/Chem3300/phyto3.pdf
55. US National Institute of Neurological Disorders and Stroke. "Brain Basics: Know Your Brain," available at http://www.ninds.nih.gov/disorders/brain_basics/know_your_brain.htm, accessed on March 20, 2012.
56. US National Institute of Neurological Disorders and Stroke,. *Headache: Hope Through Research,* available at http://www.ninds.nih.gov/disorders/headache/headachehope.pdf, accessed on March 20, 2012.
57. Gengo FM. "Pharmacological Principles in Treating Neurological Disease," in Bradley WG, Daroff RB, Fenichel GM, Janovic J. *Neurology in Clinical Practice* 5th ed. Butterworth-Heinemann, 2008.
58. Mahowald MW. "Disorders of Sleep," in Goldman L, Schafer AI, *Cecil Medicine,* 24th ed, Philadelphia, Elsevier, 2011.
59. US National Library of Medicine. "Melatonin," available at http://www.nlm.nih.gov/medlineplus/druginfo/natural/940.html, accessed on March 25, 2012.
60. The Mayo Clinic. "Depression (Major Depression): Serotonin and Norepinephrine Reuptake Inhibitors (SNRIs)," available at http://www.mayoclinic.com/health/antidepressants/MH00067, accessed on March 26, 2012.
61. US National Institutes of Health. National Institute on Drug Abuse. "Impact of Drugs on Neurotransmission," available at http://www.drugabuse.gov/news-events/nida-notes/2007/10/impacts-drugs-neurotransmission. accessed on March 26, 2012.
62. Lyness JM. "Psychiatric Disorders in Medical Practice," in Goldman L, Schafer AI, *Cecil Medicine,* 24th ed, .Philadelphia, Elsevier, 2011.
63. Charlson M, "Complementary and Alternative Medicine," in Goldman L, Schafer AI, *Cecil Medicine,* 24th ed, .Philadelphia, Elsevier, 2011.
64. American Heart Association, "Take Action to Control Stress," available at http://www.heart.org/HEARTORG/GettingHealthy/StressManagement/TakeActiontoControlStress/Take-Action-To-Control-Stress_UCM_001402_Article.jsp, accessed on March 21, 2012.
65. The Mayo Clinic.."Stress: Constant Stress Puts Your health at Risk," available at http://www.heart.org/HEARTORG/GettingHealthy/StressManagement/TakeActiontoControlStress/Take-Action-To-Control-Stress_UCM_001402_Article.jsp, accessed on March 21, 2012.
66. US National Institutes of health, National Center for Complementary and Alternative Medicine, "Tea Tree Oil," available at http://nccam.nih.gov/health/tea/treeoil.htm, accessed on March 22, 2012.
67. US National Library of Medicine, "Tea Tree Oil," available at http://www.nlm.nih.gov/medlineplus/druginfo/natural/113.html, accessed on March 22, 2012.
68. American Cancer Society, "tea Tree Oil," available at http://www.cancer.org/Treatment/TreatmentsandSideEffects/ComplementaryandAlternativeMedicine/HerbsVitaminsandMinerals/index, accessed on March 22, 2012.
69. US Food and Drug Administration, "Trans fat Now Listed with saturated Fat and Cholesterol," available at http://www.fda.gov/Food/ResourcesForYou/Consumers/NFLPM/ucm274590.htm, accessed on March 20, 2012.
70. Mayo Clinic, Trans fat is double trouble for your heart health," available at. http://www.mayoclinic.com/health/trans-fat/CL00032/METHOD=print, accessed on March 20, 2012.
71. Underbakke G, McBride PE. "Dyslipidemias," in Rakel D. *Integrative Medicine* 2nd ed. Philadelphia, Saunders, 2007.

Thoughts are like drops of water which flow down

stream to collect with other small streams, to

*collectively become a mighty river.*PH

About the Appendices: The following information is provided to complement your practice of the nine steps; the relevant step is noted for each appendix. Some of the nutrients included have been chosen due to their relatively underappreciated value, while others are more commonplace and widely recognized but of significant importance. I believe you will find useful information here for assisting in your LifeReStyle Process by following or adopting the Nine Natural Steps.

For ongoing support and information, visit:

www.StressPandemic.com and www.LifeReStyle.org

APPENDIX A

Step 5: Exercise

1. Guide To Preventing Walking Injury

- Wear well-cushioned shoes providing solid side-to-side stability. Purchase shoes after you have been walking for a while, as your feet are largest later in the day. And be sure to have both of your feet measured and if one foot is larger purchase shoes that fit your largest foot. People with high-arched, low-arch (or flat), and neutral-arched feet benefit from shoes that provide different types of support; be certain to select shoes that are right for you.

- Select comfortable, protective clothing.

- Wear bright colors or reflective tape after dark so that motorists can see you.

- Spend about five minutes walking slowly to warm up your muscles. Increase your pace until you feel warm.

- After warming up, stretch your muscles before walking. A free brochure from the US National Institutes of Health (NIH) presents stretches recommended for before and after you walk. As the NIH says, stretch gently, overdoing does not help. The brochure, "Walking... a step in the right direction," is available at http://win.niddk.nih.gov/publications/PDFs/walking2004.pdf

- The American Academy of Podiatric Sports Medicine recommends that people forty years of age and older and people with diabetes, preexisting injuries, a family history of heart problems, or any circulatory or breathing problems should check with a physician before starting to exercise.

- The American Academy of Podiatric Sports medicine states: "Psychologically, walking generates an overall feeling of well-being, and can relieve depression, anxiety, and stress by producing endorphins, the body's natural tranquilizer. A brisk walk will relax you and stimulate your thinking."

Cool down after each walking session to reduce stress on your heart and muscles; conclude each walking session by walking slowly for about five minutes. Then repeat your stretches. It is best to do your stretches up against a wall or a park bench. Try to find a natural way to exercise and stretch.

Sources:
1. American Academy of Podiatric Sports Medicine: "Walking and Your Feet: benefits of Exercise Walking," available at http://www.aapsm.org/walking.html, accessed on March 26, 2012:
2. The Maryo Clinic. "Walking Shoes: Features and Fit That Keep You Moving," available at http://www.mayoclinic.com/print/walking/HQ00885_D/METHOD=print, accessed on March 26, 2012:
3. Mader E, Bucher B. "Central pattern generators and the control of rhythmic movements." *ScienceDirect,* November27, 2001. 11(23):986-996. http://www.sciencedirect.com/science/article/pii/S0960982201005814
4. Mondal S, Nandi A. et al. "Modeling a Central Pattern Generator to Generate the Biped Locomotion of a Bipedal Robot Using Rayleigh Oscillators" Indian Institute of Information Technology. 2011. 168: 289-300. http://www.academia.edu/1952963/Modeling_a_Central_Pattern_Generator_to_Generate_the_Biped_Locomotion_of_a_Bipedal_Robot_Using_Rayleigh
5. MacKay-Lyons M. "Central Pattern Generation of Locomotion: A Review of the Evidence." *The Journal of the American Physical Therapy,* January 2002, 82: 169-83. http://physicaltherapyjournal.com/content/82/1/69.full

We can do anything we set our minds to do.
We can be anything our mind sets itself to be.
If we have true awareness,
we can have the perfect haven where we want to go.
This is the power of our amazing mind. PH

2. Breathing and Stretching Exercises

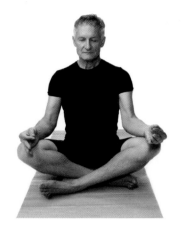

Calm heart meditation

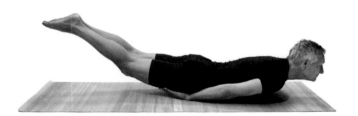

Grasshopper

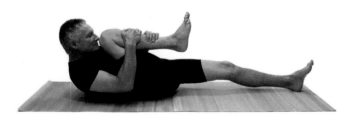

Knee to head pose

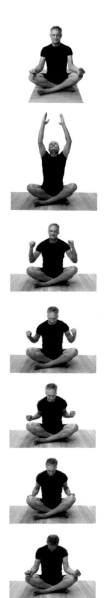

Stretching and breathing exercises are an important way to reduce stress. You can do these simple exercises anywhere; and they do not require special equipment or facilities. Refer to the instructional video on the Stress Pandemic website for the full set of exercises: www. StressPandemic.com and www. LifeReStyle.org.

Vital energy breathing

APPENDIX B
Step 6: Nutrition

1. Mercury in Fish

Mercury is a naturally occurring substance. In addition, industrial pollution leads to the release of mercury. As it accumulates in streams and oceans, mercury is transformed into methylmercury, and fish absorb methylmercury as they feed. In fish, as in humans, methylmercury can build up over time. It is notable that the human body naturally rids itself of methylmercury; however, this is a gradual process that can take more than a year.

It is a scientific fact that for people of all ages ingesting high levels of mercury can harm the brain, heart, kidneys, lungs, and immune system. It is particularly important for pregnant women and women of childbearing age who should be careful about consuming methylmercury. Yet these women, like nearly everyone else, benefit from eating fish. So what should be done? People with small children who want to use the list as a guide should reduce portion sizes.

All of us may benefit from avoiding those fish that carry high levels of mercury and, instead, looking to fish with lower levels of this substance. Fish higher in mercury include larger fish, as they have lived longer and have had time to accumulate greater levels of mercury. These include swordfish, shark, king mackerel, and tilefish.

Be aware that in the US and certain other countries, you can check online and learn about mercury levels of fish caught in local waters.

Consumer Guide to Mercury in Fish

LEAST MERCURY:

Enjoy these fish: Anchovies, Butterfish, Catfish, Clam, Crab (Domestic), Crawfish/ Crayfish, Croaker (Atlantic), Flounder*, Haddock (Atlantic)*, Hake, Herring, Mackerel (N. Atlantic, Chub), Mullet, Oyster, Perch (Ocean), Plaice, Pollock, Salmon (Canned)**, Salmon (Fresh)**, Sardine, Scallop*, Shad (American), Shrimp*, Sole (Pacific), Squid (Calamari), Tilapia, Trout (Freshwater), Whitefish, Whiting

MODERATE MERCURY:

Eat six servings or less per month: Bass (Striped, Black), Carp, Cod (Alaskan)*, Croaker (White Pacific), Halibut (Atlantic)*, Halibut (Pacific), Jacksmelt, (Silverside), Lobster, Mahi Mahi, Monkfish*, Perch (Freshwater), Sablefish, Skate*, Snapper*, Tuna (Canned chunk light), Tuna (Skipjack)*, Weakfish (Sea Trout)

HIGH MERCURY:

Eat three servings or less per month: Bluefish, Grouper*, Mackerel (Spanish, Gulf), Sea Bass (Chilean)*, Tuna (Canned Albacore), Tuna (Yellowfin)*

HIGHEST MERCURY:

Avoid eating: Mackerel (King), Marlin*, Orange Roughy*, Shark*, Swordfish*, Tilefish*, Tuna, (Bigeye, Ahi)*

* Fish in trouble! These fish are perilously low in numbers or are caught using environmentally destructive methods. To learn more, see the Monterey Bay Aquarium and the Blue Ocean Institute, both of which provide guides to fish to enjoy or avoid on the basis of environmental factors.

** Farmed Salmon may contain PCBs, chemicals with serious long-term health effects.

About the mercury-level categories: The categories on the list (least mercury to highest mercury) are determined according to the following mercury levels in the flesh of tested fish: Least mercury: Less than 0.09 ppm, Moderate mercury: From 0.09 to 0.29 ppm, High mercury: From 0.3 to 0.49 ppm, Highest mercury: More than 0.5 ppm

Sources: US Food and Drug Administration. "What Your Need to Know About Mercury in Fish and Shellfish," available at http://water.epa.gov/scitech/swguidance/ fishshellfish/outreach/upload/2004_05_24_fish_MethylmercuryBrochure.pdf. accessed on March 21, 2012.

US Environmental Protection Agency, "Mercury," available at http://www.epa.gov/ mercury/about.htm, accessed on March 22, 2012.

Environmental Protection Agency. "Fish Advisories," available at http://water.epa. gov/scitech/swguidance/fishshellfish/fishadvisories/index.cfm, accessed on March 22, 2012.

Natural Resources Defense Council. "Mercury in Fish," available at http://www. nrdc.org/health/effects/mercury/walletcard.PDF, accessed on March 22, 2012.

2. LifeReStyle GOOD-MOOD FOODS
and the 5 Important Neurochemicals in the Brain

Dopamine	Alfalfa, apples, almonds, asparagus, bananas, beans, beets, blueberries, broccoli, chicken, eggs, fava beans, fish, legumes, lettuce, peanuts, pumpkin, seaweed, sesame seeds, spinach, spirulina, tofu, turkey, watermelon, wheat germ
Endorphins	Bananas, brazil nuts, cacao (natural), brown rice pasta, chicken, grapes, grapefruit, hot chillies, oranges, nuts, pasta, St John's wort, salmon, sesame seeds, strawberries, turkey, walnuts, whole grain bread
Epinephrine (or adrenaline)	Almonds, avocados, bananas, chicken, eggs, grains, most leafy greens, lean meat, nuts, pineapple, seafood, seeds, soy bean, tofu
Norepinephrine	Avocados, bananas, blue-green algae, chicken breast, fish (shrimp, tuna, cod, haddock and lobster), legumes, lima beans, oats, wheat, pumpkin seeds, seaweed, spinach, tofu
Serotonin	African griffonia beans, bananas, basil, beans, bitter gourd (karavila), blueberries, broccoli, broccolini, brown rice, buckwheat, cacao (natural), butternut, fish, flax seeds, ginko, gotu kola, green tea, herring, kiwi, maca, mandarins, nuts, orange, parsley, pecan nut, pineapple, plantains, salmon, sardines, spinach, sweet potato, plums, tart and sour cherries, tomato, turkey, whole grains
Note: Be sure not to overdose on any of your healthy dietary changes. Rotate your portions in a balanced way.	

(Sources: Harvard University, Nutritional Sources, http://www.hsph.harvard.edu/
nutritionsource/what-should-you-eat/pyramid/
Mateljan, G,. Worlds Healthiest Foods, see reference list;
http://www.mayoclinic.com/health/nutrition-and-healthy-eating/
MY00431
Readers Digest, "Fight Back with Food." Dec, 2006, Publ: Readers Digest
Aronson, D. "Cortisol: its Role in Stress, Inflammation, and Indication
for Diet Therapy", *Today's Dietitian* (2009), 11 : 38.)

C.R.A.P.: Foods and Drinks to Avoid

The gut lining, the small intestine, has what is known as having a 'Second Brain'. It is where the neurochemical serotonin – the happy mood food, has the maximum absorption. 90-95% of the serotonin receptors are found in the 'villi' of the gut lining. In eating "GOOD-MOOD FOODS" we aid the production of serotonin needed in our body, we prevent many colonic related diseases and inflammation conditions like constipation, colitis, leaky gut and allergies caused by the immune system disrupted.

C : stands for Caffeine, a stimulant that stimulates the activation of numerous neural circuits, which causes the pituitary gland in the brain to secrete hormones that in turn cause the adrenal gland to produce more adrenaline, or epinephrine (which is a fight-flight hormone). As a result, it increases your attention level and gives your entire neurochemical system an extra burst of energy. This is exactly the effect that many coffee drinkers are looking for,[1] which remains in our system for a considerable length of time, throwing it out of balance. Caffeine is an artificial stimulant, which replaces or hijacks the neurochemical Dopamine in the middle brain. (Dopamine the neurotransmitter is metabolized and stimulates or acts on the reward-pleasure center in the brain). In time you can build a dependency on this artificial stimulant and you will crave more and more. Excessive caffeine ingestion leads to symptoms that overlap with those of many psychiatric disorders. Caffeine is implicated in the exacerbation of anxiety and sleep disorders.[2] Caffeine can cause a physical and emotional dependency, with withdrawals from caffeine beginning within one or two days.

R : stands for Refined sugar, a complex carbohydrate which acts as a toxic or poisonous substances, because the liver is taxed in the process of metabolizing it, potentially leading to insulin resistance, believed to be the underlying problem in obesity, type 2 diabetes, heart disease, and possibly many cancers.[3] Refined sugar provides calories but lacks the vitamins, minerals and fiber. It is called "empty calories" and causes weight gain. Refined sugar is a disaccharide compound made of simple molecular compounds of carbon, oxygen and hydrogen, which store energy and gives it out as it breaks down. This is the reason, when we are tired and want a sugar-fix, we are able to get it from sugar in the form of cakes, candy, ice cream and others (including honey) which belong to the "sucrose" group of carbohydrates.

Other substances to avoid are brown sugar, cane sugar and artificial sweeteners.

A : stands for Alcohol, which passes directly via osmosis from the porous digestive system into the blood vessels in minutes, the blood transports the alcohol to all parts of the body, including the brain. Alcohol affects the brain in various ways. It alters the membranes as well as their ion channels, enzymes and receptors. It binds directly to Serotonin and other receptors, which is the reason you feel 'happy and get a high'. But as the dependency becomes more, the neuron activity becomes further diminished and causes a sedative effect. Chronic consumption usually desensitizes the GABA receptors, which in time may cause alcohol withdrawals. Alcohol helps increase the release of Dopamine, which stimulates the reward-pleasure center needing more alcohol over time to get the same high.[4,5]

P : stands for Processed foods and drinks, which causes inflammation of the gut and colon. It causes colitis, leaky gut and allergies due to the disruption to the immune system in the body and it also causes the disruption of sleep patterns, blood pressure, heart disease, arthritis and other symptoms and dangers of stress.[6] When you are stressed the body and the mind has a tendency to crave sugars and fats or both. Numerous artificial additives are commonly found in processed foods and drinks. Today's processed foods and drinks may include such harmful substances as MSG, food coloring, artificial flavors, aspartame, genetically modified organisms (GMOs), and nitrates, to name only a few. Avoid processed foods and drinks. Instead choose the most natural unprocessed foods, like vegetables, fruit, nuts, grains, roots, fish and meat. Drink lots of water, natural juices, and herbal teas. Use natural oils e.g. A study published in 2010 used coconut oil to show that a diet enriched in the saturated fatty acids of coconut oil offered strong advantages for the protection against oxidative stress in heart mitochondria which function on a cellular level.[7]

Avoiding CRAP or having in strict moderation, and leaning towards a diet high in Good-Mood Foods, will enable you to obtain longevity and a healthier life.

Sources:
1. a) http://thebrain.mcgill.ca/flash/i/i_03/i_03_m/i_03_m_par/i_03_m_par_cafeine.html
   b) Caffeine – Dopamine effect – The Brain From Top To Bottom http://thebrain.mcgill.ca/flash/i/i_03/i_03_m/i_03_m_par/i_03_m_par_cafeine.html
2. Winston AP, Hardwick E, Jaberi N. "Neuropsychiatric effects of caffeine"
3. a) http://ajcn.nutrition.org/content/early/2013/06/26/ajcn.113.064113.abstract
   b) http://www.ncbi.nlm.nih.gov/pubmed/19538307?itool=EntrezSystem2.PEntrez.Pubmed.Pubmed_ResultsPanel.Pubmed_RVDocSum&ordinalpos=2
   c) http://ngm.nationalgeographic.com/2013/08/sugar/cohen-text
4. Alcohol : The Brain From Top To Bottom: http://thebrain.mcgill.ca/flash/i/i_03/i_03_m/i_03_m_par/i_03_m_par_alcool.html#drogues
5. a) Avery DH, Bolte MA, Ries R. "Dawn simulation treatment of abstinentalcoholics with winter depression." Department of Psychiatry and Behavioral Sciences, University of Washington School of Medicine, *J. Clin. Psych,* January1998, 59:1, 36-42.
   b) Adv.in Psy. Treatment. November 2005. 11: 432 439.http://apt.rcpsych.org/content/11/6/432.full3.
6. Galland L. "Do You Have Leaky Gut Syndrome?" Random House, June 1, 1998. P 384. http://www.huffingtonpost.com/leo-galland-md/do-you-have-leaky-gut-syn_b_688951.html
7. a) http://coconutoil.com/coconut-oil-alzheimers/
   b) http://ajcn.nutrition.org/content/early/2013/06/26/ajcn.113.064113.abstract
   c) http://www.thehindu.com/todays-paper/tp-national/tp-tamilnadu/beware-of-artificially-ripened-mangoes/article4635783.ece

3. Foods Rich in Calcium

Calcium and vitamin D work together for bone and tooth health. In addition, adequate calcium ensures the healthy working of such body functions as the transmission of impulses along the nerves both within the brain and throughout the body. Calcium also serves as an intracellular messenger, helps blood vessels move blood throughout the body, enables the functioning of vitamin D, aids in homeostatic regulation, and plays a role in the release of hormones and enzymes that affect almost every function in the body.

	Weight (g)	Common Measure	mg Nutrient Content per measure
Asparagus, cooked, boiled, drained	60	4 spears	14
Beet greens, cooked, boiled, drained, without salt	144	1 cup	164
Broccoli, cooked, boiled, drained, without salt	156	1 cup	62
Brussels sprouts, cooked, boiled, drained, without salt	156	1 cup	56
Cabbage, Chinese (pak-choi), cooked, boiled, drained, without salt	170	1 cup	158
Cabbage, cooked, boiled, drained, without salt	150	1 cup	72
Celery, raw	120	1 cup	48
Collards, cooked, boiled, drained, without salt	190	1 cup	266
Cowpeas (black eyes), immature seeds, cooked, boiled, drained, without salt	165	1 cup	211
Great northern beans, mature seeds, cooked, boiled, without salt	177	1 cup	120
Green snap beans, cooked, boiled, drained, without salt	125	1 cup	55
Kale, frozen, cooked, boiled, drained, without salt	130	1 cup	179
Kelp (seaweed), raw	102	1 tbsp	17
Lettuce, romaine, raw	56	1 cup	18

	Weight (g)	Common Measure	mg Nutrient Content per measure
Mustard greens, cooked, boiled, drained, without salt	140	1 cup	104
Navy beans, mature seeds, cooked, boiled, without salt	182	1 cup	126
Okra, cooked, boiled, drained, without salt	160	1 cup	123
Oranges, raw, all commercial varieties	131	1 orange	52
Oat cereal, instant, fortified, plain, prepared with water (boiling water added or microwaved)	177	1 packet	142
Fish, sardine, Atlantic, canned in oil, drained solids with bone	85.05	3 oz	325
Sesame butter, tahini, from roasted and toasted kernels (most common type)	15	1 tbsp	64
Soybeans, mature cooked, boiled, without salt	172	1 cup	175
Spinach, cooked, boiled, drained, without salt	180	1 cup	245
Squash summer, all varieties, cooked, boiled, drained, without salt	180	1 cup	49
Tofu, soft, prepared with calcium sulfate and magnesium chloride (nigari)	120	1 piece	133
Turnip greens, cooked, boiled, drained, without salt	144	1 cup	197
White beans, mature seeds, canned	262	1 cup	191

Sources: USDA National Nutrient Database for Standard Reference, Release 24, available at https://www.ars.usda.gov/SP2UserFiles/Place/12354500/Data/SR24/nutrlist/sr24a301.pdf, accessed on March 21, 2012.

Office of Dietary Supplements, National Institutes of Health. "Calcium- Quick Facts," available at http://ods.od.nih.gov/factsheets/Calcium-QuickFacts, accessed on March 25, 2012.

Weaver CM, Heaney RP. "Calcium," in Shils ME, Shike M, Ross AC, Caballero B, Cousins RJ. *Modern Nutrition* Philadelphia, Lippincott Williams & Wilkins, 2006.

4. Foods Rich in Copper

Copper functions in the body as an essential component of numerous enzymes involved in the body's organ systems. Copper is an essential ingredient in the formation of red blood cells and in the normal working of blood vessels, bones, the immune system, and the nervous system. Copper plays an essential role in the enzyme crucial for transforming tyrosine into dopamine, in the conversion of dopamine to norepinephrine, in the adrenal gland (where it serves during epinephrine production), in forming and maintaining the nervous system's myelin, and in the degradation of serotonin, norepinephrine, and dopamine.

	Weight (g)	Common Measure	mg Nutrient Content per measure
Barley, pearled, cooked	157	1 cup	0.165
Brazil nuts, dried, unblanched	28.35	1 oz (6–8 nuts)	0.494
Buckwheat flour, whole-groat	120	1 cup	0.618
Cashew nuts, dry roasted, with salt added	28.35	1 oz	0.629
Chestnuts, European, roasted	143	1 cup	0.725
Chickpeas (garbanzo beans, bengal gram, cooked), mature seeds, canned	240	1 cup	0.418
Cowpeas, common (blackeyes, crowder, southern), mature seeds, cooked, boiled, without salt	172	1 cup	0.461
Lentils, mature seeds, cooked, boiled, without salt	198	1 cup	0.497
Lima beans,, large, mature seeds, cooked, boiled, without salt	188	1 cup	0.442
Navy beans, mature seeds, cooked, boiled, without salt	182	1 cup	0.382
Potato, baked, flesh, without salt	156	1 potato	0.335

Potatoes, baked, skin, without salt	58	1 skin	0.474
Pumpkin and squash seed kernels, roasted, with salt added	28.35	1 oz (142 seeds)	0.392
Red kidney beans, mature seeds, cooked, boiled, without salt	177	1 cup	0.428
Sesame butter, tahini, from roasted and toasted kernels (most common type)	15	1 tsp	0.242
Shitake mushroom, cooked, without salt	145	1 cup	1.299
Soybeans, mature cooked, boiled, without salt	172	1 cup	0.700
Sunflower seedkernels, dry roasted, with salt added	32	¼ cup	0.586
Tomato products, canned, puree, without salt added	250	1 cup	0.718
Walnuts, English	28.35	1oz (14 halves)	0.450

Source: USDA: National Nutrient data for Standard Reference; SR17, available at http://www.nal.usda.gov/fnic/foodcomp/Data/SR17/wtrank/sr17a312.pdf, accessed on March 19, 2012.

US National Library of Medicine. "Copper in Diet," available at http://www.nlm.nih.gov/medlineplus/ency/article/002419.htm, accessed on March 25, 2012.

Gengo FM. "Pharmacological Principles in Treating Neurological Disease," in Bradley WG, Daroff RB, Fenichel GM, Janovic J. *Neurology in Clinical Practice* 5th ed. Butterworth-Heinemann, 2008.

Turnlund JR. "Copper," in Shils ME, Shike M, Ross AC, Caballero B, Cousins RJ. *Modern Nutrition* Philadelphia, Lippincott Williams & Wilkins, 2006.

5. Foods Rich in Vitamin E (alpha-tocopherol)

Vitamin E functions as an antioxidant, which means it helps protect the cells of the body from damage caused by free radicals. These free radicals appear naturally as our bodies convert food into energy. In addition, we obtain free radicals from the environment, from cigarette smoke, air pollution, and the ultraviolet light from the sun. Vitamin E also plays an important role in combating oxidative stress and is a powerful antioxidant with anti-inflammatory properties. Other ways our bodies use vitamin E are to boost the immune system to help fight off bacteria and viruses; to widen blood vessels and so reduce the chances blood clots will form; and to help several types of body cells interact with one another.

Food	Amount	Alpha-tocopherol (mg)	Gamma-tocopherol (mg)
Olive oil	1 tbsp	1.9	0.1
Soybean oil	1 tbsp	1.1	8.7
Corn oil	1 tbsp	1.9	8.2
Canola oil	1 tbsp	2.4	3.8
Safflower oil	1 tbsp	4/6	0.1
Sunflower oil	1 tbsp	5.6	0.7

Food	Weight (g)	Common Measure	Content per Measure (mg)
Almonds	28.35	1 oz (24 nuts)	7.433
Beet greens, cooked, boiled, drained, without salt	144	1 cup	2.606
Blueberries, frozen, sweetened	230	1 cup	1.196
Broccoli, cooked, boiled, drained, without salt	156	1 cup	2.262
Carrots, frozen, cooked, boiled, drained, without salt	146	1 cup	1.475

Dandelion greens, cooked, boiled, drained, without salt	105	1 cup	2.562
Hazelnuts or filberts	28.35	1 oz	4.261
Kale, frozen, cooked, boiled, drained, without salt	130	1 cup	1.196
Kiwifruit, green, raw	76	1 medium	1.110
Lima beans, immature seeds, frozen, baby, cooked, boiled, drained, without salt	180	1 cup 1.152	
Mangos, raw 165	1 cup	1.485	
Peaches, raw	170	1 cup	1.241
Peanuts, all types, dry-roasted, with salt	28.35	1 oz (approx 28)	2.211
Pine nuts, dried	28.35	1 oz	2.645
Spinach, cooked, boiled, drained, without salt	180	1 cup	3.744
Sunflower seed kernels, dry roasted, with salt added	28.35	1 oz	7.399
Sweet potato, cooked, boiled, without skin	156	1 potato	1.466
Tomato products, canned, puree, without salt added	250	1 cup	4.925
Turnip greens, cooked, boiled, drained, without salt	144	1 cup	2.707

Source: Office of Dietary Supplements, US National Institutes of Health, "Vitamin E," available at http://ods.od.nih.gov/factsheets/VitaminE-QuickFacts/, accessed on March 23, 2012.

Linus Pauling Institute at Oregon State University. "Vitamin E," available at http://lpi.oregonstate.edu/infocenter/vitamins/vitaminE/index.html. accessed on March 23, 2012.

USDA National Nutrient Database for Standard Reference, Release 23. "Vitamin E (alpha tocopherol) (ng) Content of Selected Foods per Common Measure, sorted by nutrient content," available at http://www.ars.usda.gov/SP2UserFiles/Place/12354500/Data/SR23/nutrlist/sr23w323.pdf, accessed on March 23, 2012.

Traber MG. "Vitamin E", in Shils ME, Shike M, Ross AC, Caballero B, Cousins RJ. *Modern Nutrition Philadelphia*, Lippincott Williams & Wilkins, 2006.

6. Foods Rich in Magnesium

Magnesium plays an important role in more than 300 biochemical reactions in the human body. Normal nerve function and normal muscle activity crucially depend upon magnesium levels, as does a healthy heart rhythm and a healthy immune system. Magnesium is used by the body in the production and transport of energy, in the working of certain enzymes, in the contraction and relaxation of muscles, in the production of protein, in maintaining normal blood pressure, and in regulating blood sugar levels. While about half of all the body's magnesium is located in bone and most of the other half in body tissues and organs, the roughly one percent of the body's magnesium that is circulating in the blood is also very important. (Research shows magnesium deficiencies have been linked to depression.) Fortunately, having too much magnesium is rarely a problem (unless magnesium supplements are taken), as the body removes excess amounts.

Food	Weight (g)	Common Measure	Content per Measure (mg)
Almonds	28.35	1 oz (24 nuts)	78
Artichokes, (globe or french), cooked, boiled, drained, without salt	168	1 cup	101
Barley, pearled, raw	200	1 cup	158
Beet greens, cooked, boiled, drained, without salt	144	1 cup	98
Black beans, mature seeds, cooked, boiled, without salt	172	1 cup	120
Brazilnuts, dried, unblanched	28.35	1 oz (6-8 nuts)	107
Buckwheat flour, whole-groat	120	1 cup	301
Buckwheat groats, roasted, cooked	168	1 cup	86
Bulgur, dry	140	1 cup	230

Cashew nuts, oil roasted, with salt added	28.35	1 oz (18 nuts)	77
Chickpeas (garbanzo beans, bengal gram), mature seeds,			
boiled, without salt	164	1 cup	79
Cornmeal, whole-grain, yellow	122	1 cup	155
Cowpeas, common (blackeyes, crowder, southern), mature seeds,			
cooked, boiled, without salt	172	1 cup	91
Grapefruit juice, white, frozen concentrate, unsweetened, undiluted	207	6-fl-oz can	79
Dates, deglet noor	178	1 cup	77
Lima beans, large, mature seeds, cooked, boiled, without salt	188	1 cup	81
Kidney beans, red, mature seeds, cooked, boiled, without salt	177	1 cup	80
Navy beans, mature seeds, cooked, boiled, without salt	182	1 cup	96
Oat bran, raw	94	1 cup	221
Okra, frozen, cooked, boiled, drained, without salt	184	1 cup	94
Orange juice, frozen concentrate, unsweetened, undiluted	213	6-fl-oz can	72
Pinto beans, mature seeds, cooked, boiled, without salt	171	1 cup	86
Pumpkin seeds squash seed kernels, roasted, with salt added	28.35	1 oz (142 seeds)	151
Rice, brown, long-grain, cooked	195	1 cup	84
Spinach, cooked, boiled, drained, without salt	180	1 cup	157

Wheat flour, whole-grain	120	1 cup	166
Soybeans, mature cooked, boiled, without salt	172	1 cup	148
Tomato products, canned, paste, without salt added	262	1 cup	110
White beans, mature seeds, canned	262	1 cup	134

Source: USDA National Nutrient Database for Standard Reference, Release 18: magnesium, Mg (mg) Content of Selected Foods per Common Measure, sorted by nutrient content.," available at http://www.nal.usda.gov/fnic/foodcomp/Data/SR18/nutrlist/sr18w304.pdf, accessed on March 23, 2012.

US National Library of Medicine. "Magnesium in Diet," available at http://www.nlm.nih.gov/medlineplus/ency/article/002423.htm, accessed on March 26, 2012.

Rude RK, Shils ME. "Magnesium", in Shils ME, Shike M, Ross AC, Caballero B, Cousins RJ. *Modern Nutrition* Philadelphia, Lippincott Williams & Wilkins, 2006.

7. Foods Rich in Vitamin B, C, D and E

Vitamin	Food Sources
Vitamins B6 and B12 help maintain nervous tissues and assist in the synthesis of neurotransmitters; aid many enzymes in the metabolism of proteins and amino acids; participate in the creation of hemoglobin; assist in immune system functioning; and modulate steroid activity. Animal studies demonstrate that serotonin activity is sensitive to B6 status. As to B12, deficiency in this vitamin is associated with neurologic and psychiatric manifestations. B6 and B12 are very important for maintaining the neuronal system and tissue regeneration, cardiovascular system, the digestive tract, bone marrow regeneration and the immune system. Regeneration of collagen is important for highly active people to maintain their system.	Bananas, beans and peas, bell pepper, chicken breast, eggs, leafy green vegetables, salmon (cooked), snapper (cooked), spinach, tuna, turkey, turnip greens, whole grains (including wheat and oats)
Vitamin C is a protective antioxidant. In addition it is active in reactions required for reducing byproducts of copper or iron. There are yet additional functions of vitamin C that have yet to be elucidated, as this vitamin appears in certain specific body tissues for purposes that scientists still have been unable to account for. Vitamin C also reduces cortisol level and repairs and improves tissue growth. It cannot be stored in the body but vital for the tissue growth and repairs of the body. It is important in the formation of collagen which is needed for blood vessels, tendons, ligaments and bones. It has beneficial effects on the common cold, cancer, the aging process and the synthesis of the neurotransmitter norepinepherine which effects the mood. It reduces cortisol and the psychological stress in people.	Asparagus, beet greens, bell pepper, blueberries, broccoli, brussels sprouts, cabbage, cantaloupe, cauliflower, collard, kale, kiwifruit, lemon juice, melon, mustard greens, oranges and other citrus fruits, papaya, parsley, peaches, peas, peppers (red and green), potatoes, spinach, star fruit, strawberries, tomatoes

Vitamin	Food Sources
Vitamin D plays a role in bone and tooth health, as well as in the maintaining both intracellular and extracellular concentrations of both calcium and phosphorus. Lack of Vitamin D has always been found among the elderly and the housebound. Deficiency of Vitamin D is related to higher rates of breast, ovary, colon, and prostate cancer; increased incidence of multiple sclerosis, progression of osteoarthritis, impairment of the immune response, high blood pressure, fatigue, mood disorders (SAD), including serious depression, Type 1 diabetes and tuberculosis. Lack of Vitamin D appears to be a prime factor in the rising incidence of depression along with a lack of omega-3 fatty acids. Patients with Parkinson's disease, multiple sclerosis, congestive heart failure, and Alzheimer's disease have all been found to have significant deficits of Vitamin D. One of the main routes for ultraviolet light to be received by the body is through the eye as well as the skin.	Black beans, dates, egg yolks, fish, mature seeds, mushrooms (shiitake), salmon (cooked), turkey And, of course, sunlight* exposure permits the human body to create vitamin D. (*Sunlight is not a food source, but a good source.)
Vitamin E is an antioxidant and a scavenger of free radicals. It functions in conjunction with selenium and other antioxidants. In addition it modifies the body's processing of lipids.	Egg yolks, leafy green vegetables, vegetable oils (sunflower, canola, olive), nuts and seeds, wheat germ, whole grains (including wheat and oats)

Sources: Noel MB, Thompson M, Wadland WC, Holtrop JS. "Nutrition and Family Medicine," in Rakel RE, Pakel DP. *Textbook of Family Medicine* 8th ed. Philadelphia, Saunders, 2011.

Mason JB. Vitamins, Trace Minersls, and Other Micronutrients," in Goldman L, Schafer AI. *Cecil Medicine* 24th ed. Philadelphia, Elsevier, 2011.

Nemours Foundation, "Kids Health: Vitamins," available at http://kidshealth.org/kid/stay_healthy/food/vitamin.html, accessed on March 21, 2012.

Mackey AD, Davis SR, Gregory JF III. "Vitamin B6," in Shils ME, Shike M, Ross AC, Caballero B, Cousins RJ. *Modern Nutrition* Philadelphia, Lippincott Williams & Wilkins, 2006.

Carmel R. "Cobalamin (Vitamin B12)", in Shils ME, Shike M, Ross AC, Caballero B, Cousins RJ. Modern Nutrition Philadelphia, Lippincott Williams & Wilkins, 2006.

Levine M, Katz A, Padayatty SJ. "Vitamin C," in Shils ME, Shike M, Ross AC, Caballero B, Cousins RJ. *Modern Nutrition* Philadelphia, Lippincott Williams & Wilkins, 2006.

Holick MF. "Vitamin D," ," in Shils ME, Shike M, Ross AC, Caballero B, Cousins RJ. *Modern Nutrition* Philadelphia, Lippincott Williams & Wilkins, 2006.

8. (a) The LifeReStyle Solution Nutritional Pyramid

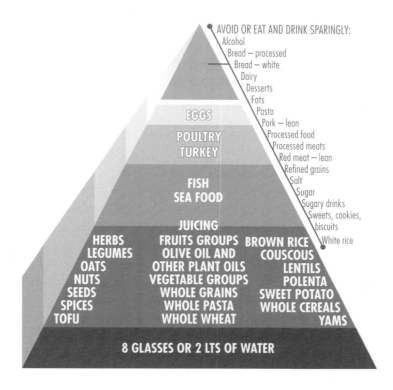

Eating is always a decision,
nobody forces your hand to pick up the food
and put it in your mouth.
Albert Ellis, Michael Abrams, Linda Dengelga,
(The Art and Science of Rational Eating).

(b) The LifeReStyle Solution Vegetarian Pyramid

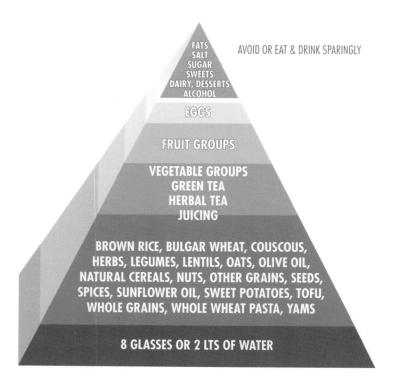

*Nothing will benefit human health
and increase the chances for survival of life on earth
as much as the evolution to a vegetarian diet.*
Albert Einstein

9. The LifeReStyle Solution Glycemic Index Food Chart

Using the glycemic index, you can quickly see how much a given food boosts blood sugar. Diets with lots of foods high on the glycemic index have been linked to diabetes, heart disease, and overweight. The University of Sydney, Australia, makes available to the public a searchable database at www.glycemicindex that currently includes more than 1,500 entries.

The following chart presents information in a handy form:

LOW	MEDIUM	HIGH
GI – 55 and under	**GI – 56 to 69**	**GI – 70 and above**
VEGETABLES		
Artichokes, asparagus, aubergine, baby marrow, brinjals, broccoli, brussel sprouts, butter nut (cooked), cabbage, carrots, celery, capsicum (peppers), cauliflower, cucumber, courgettes, eggplants, green beans, leeks, lettuce, mushrooms, okra, onions, peas, radishes, rocket, spinach, spring onions, squash, swiss chard (silver beet), tomato, zucchini	Avocado, beetroot, bean sprouts, bok choy, chard, chives, chilies, corn, endives, fennel, garlic, ginger, herbs, shallot, snow peas, sprouts, sweet corn, sweet potatoes, taro, turnips, watercress, yams	Broad beans, parsnips, potatoes, pumpkin
FRUITS		
Apples, blackberries, blueberries, cherries, cranberries (dried), figs (dried), grapefruit, gooseberries, grapes (white), guava, kiwifruits, lemons, limes, mandarins, mangoes, nectarines, oranges, prunes (dried), peaches (dried), pears, plums, rhubarb, strawberries, tangelo	Apricots, bananas, currants, dates, melon, papaya, raisins, raspberries, sultanas	Figs, grapes (black), lychee, pawpaw, pineapple, raisins, rockmelon, watermelon

LOW	MEDIUM	HIGH
GI – 55 and under	**GI – 56 to 69**	**GI – 70 and above**
LEGUMES		
Baked beans, black beans, black eyed peas, borlotti beans, butter beans, cannelloni beans, chickpeas, garbanzo beans, kidney beans, lentils (green & red), red kidney beans, lima beans, lmbo beans, mung beans, navy beans (haricot), pinto beans, speckled beans, split peas, soybeans, white beans		Broad beans
BREAD & FLOUR		
Chickpea flour (hummus), coarse barley bread, corn tortilla, oat bran flour, pumpernickel bread, rice bran flour, soy flour, split pea flour (dal), wheat bran flour, whole grain bread, whole wheat tortilla	Buckwheat flour, oats, pita bread, quinoa flour, rye flour	Most breads
CEREALS		
Allbran, rolled oats, oat bran, semolina, khorasan, soy porridge, rice bran	Oatmeal, muesli, raisin bran, Special K	Many cereals have a high GI
GRAINS, RICE & PASTA		
Brown rice, bulgur, buckwheat, cassava (cooked), pearled barley, quinoa, sweet corn on the cob, soba noodles, vermicelli, whole wheat kernels, whole wheat pasta, wild rice	Basmati rice, brown long grained rice, buck wheat noodles, cous cous, gnocchi	Amaranth, millet, rice puffs, tapioca
JUICE		
Apple, cranberry, grapefruit, orange, tomato		

- Low GI diets help people lose and manage weight
- Low GI diets increase the body's sensitivity to insulin
- Low GI carbs improve diabetes management
- Low GI carbs reduce the risk of heart disease
- Low GI carbs improve blood cholesterol levels
- Low GI carbs can help you manage the symptoms of PCOS
- Low GI carbs reduce hunger and keep you fuller for longer
- Low GI carbs prolong physical endurance

High GI carbs help refuel carbohydrate stores after exercise

How to Switch to a Low GI Diet

The basic and simplified technique for eating the low GI way is simply a "this for that" approach, swapping low GI carbs for high GI carbs.

- Use breakfast cereals based on oats, barley, bran
- Use breads from wholegrains, stone-ground flour, sourdough
- Reduce the amount of potatoes you eat
- Enjoy all other types of fruit and vegetables
- Use Basmati, Doongara or brown rice
- Enjoy whole wheat pasta, rice noodles, quinoa
- Eat plenty of salad vegetables with a vinaigrette dressing

Sources: Glycemic Index Foundation (website), available at http://www.gifoundation. com/, accessed on March 28, 2012.

Mahan LK, Escott-Stump S, Raymond JL. *Krause's Food & the Nutrition Care Process* 13th ed. Philadelphia, Elsevier, 2012.

Mahan LK, Escott-Stump S. *Krause's Food, Nutrition and Diet* 10th ed. Philadelphia, Saunders, 2000.

The University of Sydney. "Search for the Glycemic Index," available at http://www. glycemicindex.com/, accessed on March 28, 2012.

The Mayo Clinic. "Glycemic Index Diet: What's Behind the Claims," available at http://www.mayoclinic.com/health/glycemic-index-diet/MY00770, accessed on March 28, 2012.

Harvard School of Public Health. "Carbohydrates: Good Carbs Guide the Way," available at http://www.hsph.harvard.edu/nutritionsource/what-should-you-eat/carbohydrates-full-story/index.html#glycemic-index, accessed on March 28, 2012.

Harvard Health Publications: Harvard Medical School. "Glycemic Index and Glycemic Load for 100+ foods," available at http://www.health.harvard.edu/newsweek/Glycemic_index_and_glycemic_load_for_100_foods.htm, accessed on March 28, 2012.

10. Protein

Is a macro nutrient composed of amino acids that is necessary for the proper growth and function of the human body.

- Alfalfa
- Almonds
- Avocado
- Barley
- Black beans
- Blue green algae
- Broccoli
- Cashew nuts
- Chard
- Chicken Breast
- Dark leafy Greens
- Egg white
- Fava beans
- Fish
- Flax seeds
- Kidney beans
- Lean meat, Crab & Lobster (sparingly)
- Lentils
- Lima beans
- Mung beans
- Nuts and seeds :
- Oats
- Peanuts
- Pecans
- Pine nuts
- Pistachios
- Pumpkins
- Sea Vegetables/Sea Weed
- Sesame flower
- Soy protein, Tempeh, Mature Soy beans
- Spinach
- Spirulina
- Split peas
- Squash
- Sun flower seeds
- Tofu
- Turkey Breast
- Walnuts
- Watercress
- Watermelon seeds

Protein is necessary for the building and repair of body tissues. It produces enzymes, hormones, and other substances the body uses.

It regulates body processes, such as water balancing, transporting nutrients, and making muscles contract.

It keeps the body healthy by resisting diseases that are common to malnourished people and prevents one from becoming easily fatigued by producing stamina and energy.

It is found in muscles, bone, hemoglobin, myoglobin, hormones, antibodies, and enzymes, and makes up about 45% of the human body. Muscle is approximately 70% water and only about 20% protein.

http://www3.georgetown.edu/admin/auxiliarysrv/dining/nutrition/protein.html

USDA National Nutrient Database for Standard Reference. Release 15. http://www.nal.usda.gov/fnic/foodcomp/Data/SR15/wtrank/sr15a203.pdf

USDA National Nutrient Database for Standard Reference. Release 18. http://www.nal.usda.gov/fnic/foodcomp/Data/SR18/nutrlist/sr18a203.pdf

National Nutrient Database for Standard Reference
Release 25 Basic Report
Nutrient data for 11445, Seaweed, kelp, raw
http://ndb.nal.usda.gov/ndb/foods/show/3289?fg=&man=&lfacet=&count=&max=&sort=&qlookup=&offset=&format=Full&new=

Note: There are many sources of protein

Good-Mood Food
is nature's magical healer
*at its best.*PH

11. Antioxidants

The total antioxidant capacity of the foods does not necessarily reflect their health benefit. Benefits depend on how the food's antioxidants are absorbed and utilized in the body to defend itself against oxidative stress, which occurs on a cellular level. This chart should help you add more antioxidants to their daily diet.

Rank	Food item	Serving size	Total antioxidant capacity per serving
1	Small Red Bean (dried)	Half cup	13,727
2	Wild blueberry	1 cup	13,427
3	Red kidney bean (dried)	Half cup	13,259
4	Pinto bean	Half cup	11,864
5	Blueberry (cultivated)	1 cup	9,019
6	Cranberry	1 cup (whole)	8,983
7	Artichoke (cooked)	1 cup (hearts)	7,904
8	Blackberry	1 cup	7,701
9	Prune	Half cup	7,291
10	Raspberry	1 cup	6,058
11	Strawberry	1 cup	5,938
12	Red Delicious apple	1 whole	5,900
13	Granny Smith apple	1 whole	5,381
14	Pecan	1 ounce	5,095
15	Sweet cherry	1 cup	4,873
16	Black plum	1 whole	4,844
17	Russet potato (cooked)	1 whole	4,649
18	Black bean (dried)	Half cup	4,181
19	Plum	1 whole	4,118
20	Gala apple	1 whole	3,903

1) http://www.webmd.com/food-recipes/20-common-foods-most-antioxidants
2) http://lpi.oregonstate.edu/f-w00/flavonoid.html
3) http://www.sciencedaily.com/releases/2004/06/040617080908.htm
4) http://ndb.nal.usda.gov

APPENDIX C
Step 7: Sleep

Required Hours of Sleep

AGE	SLEEP NEEDED
Newborns (0 to 2 months)	12–18 hours
Infants (3 months to 1 year)	14–15 hours
Toddlers (1 to 3 years)	12–14 hours
Preschoolers (3 to 5 years)	11–13 hours
School-aged children (5 to 12 years)	10–11 hours
Teens and preteens (12 to 18 years)	8.5–10 hours
Adults (18 years +)	7.5–9 hours

(Source: http://www.sleepforkids.org/html/practices.html.)

Hyponogram of Sleep

The periods of NREM and REM sleep alternate during the night. Second, the deepest stages of NREM sleep occur in the first part of the night. Third, the episodes of REM sleep are longer as the night progresses. This hypnogram also indicates two periods during the night when the individual awakened (at about six and seven hours into the night).

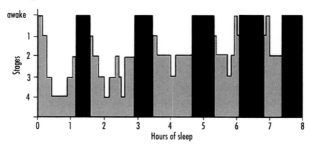

A typical hypnogram from a young, healthy adult.
Light-gray areas represent non–rapid eye movement (NREM) sleep.

Comparison of Physiological Changes During NREM and REM Sleep

Physiological Process	During NREM	During REM
Brain activity	Decreases from wakefulness	Increases in motor and sensory areas, while other areas are similar to NREM
Heart rate	Slows from wakefulness	Increases and varies compared with NREM
Blood pressure	Decreases from wakefulness	Increases (up to 30 percent) and varies from NREM
Blood flow to brain	Does not change from wakefulness in most regions	Increases by 50 to 200 percent from NREM, depending on brain region
Respiration	Decreases from wakefulness	Increases and varies from NREM, but may show brief stoppages (apnea); coughing suppressed
Airway resistance	Increases from wakefulness	Increases and varies from wakefulness
Body temperature	Is regulated at lower set point than wakefulness; shivering initiated at lower temperature than during wakefulness	Is not regulated; no shivering or sweating; temperature drifts toward that of the local environment
Sexual arousal	Occurs infrequently	Increases from NREM (in both males and females)

(Source: National Institute of Health: National Center on Sleep Disorder Research:http://science.education.nih.gov/supplements/nih3/sleep/guide/info-sleep.htm.)

APPENDIX D

Foot Reflexology

Activities such as walking barefoot can stimulate the 7200 nerve endings in the feet.

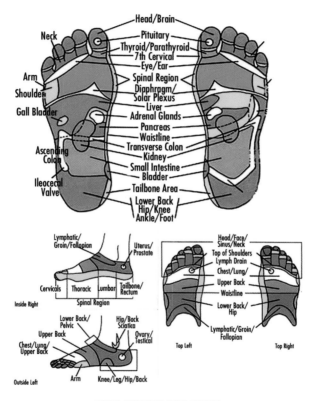

FOOT REFLEXOLOGY CHART
© 1980 Kevin and Barbara Kunz, authors of
The Complete Guide to Foot Reflexology, Revised
and other books about reflexology.

APPENDIX E

Additional Lifestyle Solution Benefits

There are many ways to manage stress. I have not covered all of them in this book. Through experimentation and discovery, find the combination of stress-reducing practices that works best for you. You will find further information about the topics below at www.StressPandemic.com and www.LifeReStyle.org.

- Acupuncture & acupressure
- Body detoxification
- Crystal Therapy
- Massage
- Light therapy
- Music & dance therapy
- Oral detoxification
- Reflexology
- Steam & sauna
- Painting
- Swimming

Three things cannot be long hidden:

the sun, the moon, and the truth.

Siddartha Gauthama

APPENDIX F

Neurochemistry and The Stress Response

The LifeReStyle NEUROCHEMISTRY and The Stress Response.

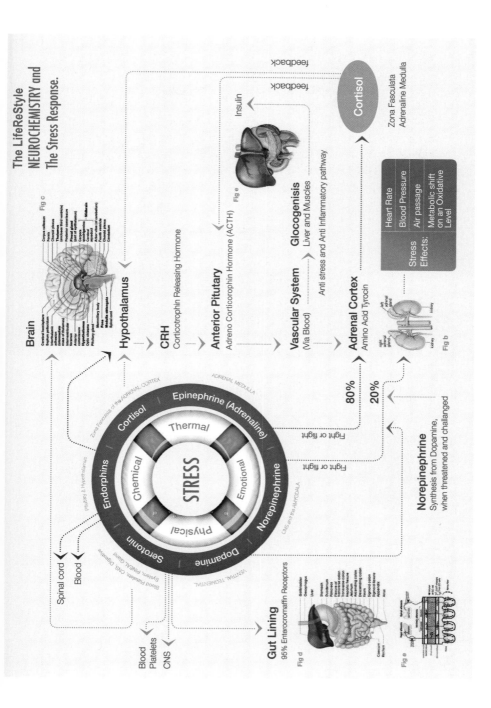

Brain Fig c

Hypothalamus

CRH Corticotrophin Releasing Hormone

Anterior Pituitary Adreno Corticorophin Hormone (ACTH)

Vascular System (Via Blood)

Glocogenisis Liver and Muscles

Anti stress and Anti Inflammatory pathway

Adrenal Cortex Amino Acid Tyrocin

Fig b

Cortisol
Zona Fasculata
Adrenaline Medulla

Insulin

feedback
feedback

Fig e

Stress Effects:	Heart Rate
	Blood Pressure
	Air passage
	Metabolic shift on an Oxidative Level

STRESS

ZONA FRACULATA of the ADRENAL CORTEX
ADRENAL MEDULLA

Cortisol / Epinephrine (Adrenaline)
Thermal
Chemical — Emotional
Endorphins
Physical
Serotonin — Dopamine — Norepinephrine

Pituitary & Hypothalamus
CNS and the AMYGDALA
VENTRAL TEGMENTAL System, PINEAL Gland
Blood Platelets CNS Objective

80%
20%
Fight or flight
Fight or flight

Norepinephrine
Synthesis from Dopamine, when threatened and challanged

Spinal cord
Blood

Blood Platelets
CNS

Gut Lining
95% Enterocromaffin Receptors

Fig d

Fig e

NEUROCHEMISTRY and The Stress Response.

(A) Serotonin (5HT) – (Fig a,d,e – page 323)

Seratonin chemical formula C10 H12N2 O. It is a neurotransmitter found throughout the body, with only a relatively small amount found in the brain. Serotonin cannot cross the blood-brain barrier. Therefore serotonin that is used inside the brain must be produced within it. Serotonin is found in the lumen of the digestive tract (GI), the central nervous system(CNS), blood platelets and the pineal gland (deep at the center of the brain). It is also known as 5-hydroxytryptamine, which is often abbreviated to 5HT. [http://www.medicalnewstoday.com/articles/232248.php]

Serotonin is also thought to be a neurohormone, a substance in our body that regulates and controls the activity of certain cells and organs. [http://onlinelibrary.wiley.com/doi/10.1111/j.1749-6632.1962.tb50107.x/abstract]. When serotonin is released into the space between neurons, it diffuses over a relatively wide gap (>20um) to activate the 5-HT receptors located in the dendrite where the cell bodies and presynaptic terminals of adjacent neurons set of a reaction. Serotonin is carried throughout the body in the blood platelets, from where it is metabolized mainly in the liver, and oxidized and extracted by the kidney. It also finds it way out of the tissue into the blood, where it is actively taken up by the blood platelets and stored. When disgorged, it acts a vasoconstrictor and regulates hemostasis and blood clotting, which is important in healing of wounds when in trauma.

About 80%- 95% of our body's total serotonin is in the "gut lining", in the enterochromaffin cells, in the villi of the gastrointestinal tract (GI), where it regulates intestinal movements. The rest is synthesized in the serotonergic neurons in the central nervous system (CNS). It is a chemical substance that transmits impulses across spaces, which are called "synapses". It is the space between nerve cells or "Ergic neurons" in the CNS. It referred to the serotonergic action outside of the CNS – causing contraction of smooth muscle. Yet, within the central nervous system, it involves other functions such as arousal, thermoregulation, mood, appetite, sleep and pain regulatory systems. An imbalance or alteration of serotonin may influence mood and lead to depression, lack of intimacy and romance, loss of instinct. It causes vasoconstriction which results in sleep issues, migraine, vomiting, anxiety, memory and learning issues. Lack of serotonin diminishes appetite, sexual behavior and suppresses pain perception. Its absence has been correlated with an increase of aggressive behavior. There is a strong correlation between serotonin levels and aggression. [http://www.macalester.edu/academics/psychology/whathap/ubnrp/placebo/serotonin2.html]

When the seasons change, and there is less sunlight, the transportation of serotonin carrying protein molecules is lower around the brain. This makes a person 'miserable', resulting in a condition known as SAD (Seasonal Addictive Disorder). http://www.european-hospital.com/en/article/4419-Seasonal_mood_changes_visualised_by_PET.html

(B) Epinephrine (Adrenaline) (Fig b – page 323)

Epinephrine chemical formula is, 4,5-β-trihydroxy-N-methylphenethylamine. It is a neurotransmitter and a hormone. They are adrenomedullary hormones; catecholamines secreted from the adrenal medulla

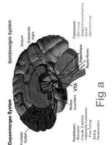

Fig a

by chromaffin cells, or neurosecretory cells, which are connected to the central nervous system. It is synthesized in the Adrenal Medulla. Adrenal glands, which are also called suprarenal glands', are small, triangular glands located on top of each kidney. An adrenal gland is made of two parts. The outer region is called the adrenal cortex and the inner region is called the adrenal medulla. Adrenaline gland via the enzymatic pathway, converts Amino Acid Tyrosine to Adrenaline. Adrenal glands work interactively with the hypothalamus and pituitary gland in the brain. For example, for the adrenal gland to produce corticosteroid hormones: the hypothalamus needs to produces corticotrophin-releasing hormone (CRH) that stimulates the pituitary gland to produce adrenocorticotropic hormone (ACTH). This ACTH stimulates the adrenal glands to make and release corticosteroid hormones, which is released into the blood.

The adrenal medulla (the inner part of the adrenal gland) helps a person cope with physical and emotional stress. The adrenal medulla secretes the following hormones:

Epinephrine (is also called adrenaline). This hormone helps the body to respond to a stressful situation, by reacting to the fight-or-flight response, by increasing the heart rate and the force of heart contractions, blood vessels, air passage (relaxation of the smooth muscle in the airways, contraction of muscles in the arterioles), cardiac arrest, facilitates blood flow to the muscles and brain, causes relaxation of smooth muscles, helps with conversion of glycogen to glucose in the liver, and other physiological changes like asthma, anaphylaxis, superficial bleeding, hair standing on end, croup, even tiredness, falling asleep and difficulty in waking up in the morning. A person may have salt or sugar cravings or be stimulated by a need for caffeine to get through the day

There is a link between adrenaline and anger, and mood change, due to the activity in the aggression center. [http://psych.gr/documents/psychiatry/15.2-EN-89.pdf]

Adrenaline Fatigue Syndrome (AFS), is when the adrenaline glands have an inability to produce enough adrenaline hormones to supply the demands of the kidney. (Not Addison's disease").

(C) Norepinephrine (Noradrenaline) (Fig b,c – page 323)

Norepinephrine is a neurotransmitter which has multiple roles, as a neurotransmitter and a hormone. It is very important for vigilance and concentration. Areas that produce norepinephrine or are effected by it, in the body are termed "Noradrenergic". Noradrenaline is produced by nerve cells and secreted into the circulation. It is a substance in our body that is produced to regulate and control the activity of certain cells or organs.

It is released from the Central Nervous System (CNS) to the sympathetic neurons in the nervous system to have a direct effect on the heart. It is synthesized from the dopamine in the secretory glands, of the neuroendocrine cells or chromaffin cells found in the medulla of the adrenal gland (above the Kidney).

• This hormone has little effect on smooth muscle, metabolic processes, and cardiac output, but does have strong vasoconstrictive effects, thus increasing blood pressure in response to acute stress.

• It is also a stress related hormone, that effects the Amygdala in the brain, to increase neuronal energy and activity, thereby controls the attention and response of the Fight or Flight response (together Adrenaline), to increase the heart rate, blood flow to skeletal muscle, increase oxygen to the brain and decreases or suppresses neuroinflammation.

All body tissue have 'adrenergic receptors'. When there is a metabolic shift in the body, it causes a Fight-or-Flight reaction.

[http://www.hopkinsmedicine.org/healthlibrary/conditions/endocrinology/adrenal_glands_85,P00399]

(D) Dopamine – (Fig a)

Dopamine chemical composition is contracted from 3,4-dihydroxyphenethylamine, a monoamine (-NH2). It is a neurotransmitter and a hormone (DOPA: Dihydroxyphenyle alanise) that is found in the brains 'Dopamine Pathways'. Dopamine functions as a neurotransmitter in the brain, releasing chemicals which send signals to other nerve cells, which connects with five dopamine nerve receptors in the human brain. It stimulates D1-D2-D3-D4-D5, found in several areas of the brains 'substantia nigra' and 'ventral tegmentia' area. They play different roles in motivation, one of which is very important in stimulating the reward motivational and pleasure center and some dopamine is important in the motor control of the nervous system.

Dopamine is produced in response to stress, and plays a major role in the Reward-Driven Learning. Every reward increases the dopamine transmission to the brain, where it 'hijacks' the natural reward system. Reward and reinforcement can frequently be used interchangeably.

When the dopamine is high in the brain, it causes an addiction, to drugs (prescription or recreational), stimulants, cocaine, methamphetamines, alcohol, smoking, sex, or even a child or adult being addicted to the internet or have disordered personality traits e.g. extraversions are linked to higher sensitivity (by stimulating the reward stimulus of the mesolimbic dopamine). The dysfunction of the dopamine system, also causes the reduction of dopamine release to the substantia nigra, which is the cause of Parkinson's disease: a degenerative disease which causes tremor and motor impairment. Restless Leg Syndrome (RLS), ADHD and with some evidence to support schizophrenia is due to some altered levels of dopamine. http://www.neuroscience.cam.ac.uk/research/cameos/AddictedBrain.php

Dopamine functions in all parts of the body, on blood vessels, inhibits norepinephrine release, acts as a chemical messenger, on the kidney, to increase sodium excretion in urine, and reduces the insulin production in the pancreas. It reduces the gastrointestinal mobility, protects intestinal mucus, and protects the immune system and the interaction between the nervous system which may cause some auto-immune conditions. It is produced locally, and exerts it effects to the closest cells. http://wings.buffalo.edu/aru/MALTA.html

(E) Endorphins – "endogenous morphine" – (Fig c – page 323)

Endorphins is a class which has 5 compounds that includes α-endorphin, β-endorphin, γ-endorphin, α-neo-endorphin, and β-neo-endorphin. A peptide with a sequence of 31 or more amino acids. They are produced by the central nervous system (CNS) and the pituitary gland. They are endogenous opioids and inhibitory neuropeptides. Endorphins are released when nerve impulses reach the spinal cord. It is released to prevent nerve cells from releasing more pain signals.

Endorphins are neurotransmitters, which are released into the blood stream from the pituitary gland into the spinal cord, and the brain from the hypothalamus. It is an endogenous 'opioid peptide' that functions as a endorphin. The main receptors are the Theta-Opioids. They disinhibit the Dopamine Pathway, causing more dopamine to be released by hijacking the process. Opioids causes inappropriate dopamine release, which causes a dependency. For example a "Runners High", is where a runner can keep running despite pain, or when a person is over the threshold by doing strenuous and continuous workout or exercise, and the person experiences moderate to high breathing difficulties, this would activate the endorphin production to ease the pain, where a person may pass the pain threshold, and the body bypass the physical limits, to be exposed to bodily harm from stress. During strenuous bodily functioning, e.g. during exercise the muscles use up stored glycogen, and release endorphins to overcome pain. The pain receptors, the 'opioid receptors' have many functions. They are a endogenous morphine – a painkiller. They act when there is excess excitement, pain, consumption of hot and spicy foods, orgasm,

cardiac, gastric, vascular functions, panic, satiation(satisfy), depersonalization disorder (a mental condition, where the person is physically not occupying the body and not in control of there speech), acupuncture or pregnancy (a fetus at 3 months makes the mother endorphin dependent). http://www.ncbi.nlm.nih.gov/pmc/articles/PMC3104618/

A term "endorphin rush" is a feeling brought on by pain, danger, or other forms of stress.

(F) Cortisol – (Fig b – page 323)

Cortisol is a hydrocortisone steroid hormone that is the most important human glucocorticoid. It is produced and released into the blood stream and the vascular system from the zona fasiculata in the adrenal cortex, which is triangular shaped organ, which sits on top of the two kidneys. It is the second layer above the adrenal cortex.

When stimulated in response to stress, and low levels of blood glucocorticoids, it causes the brain's hypothalamus to release CRH (corticotrophin hormone), which in turn causes the anterior pituitary, through a 'feedback system' to release ACTH (Adrenocorticotrophin Hormone) back to the vascular system. Its function is to increase the blood sugar through gluconeogenesis, which is the formation of glucose in the liver and stored in muscles at a natural level of a balanced body. It suppresses the immune system, and aid the metabolism of protein, fat, and carbohydrate. It also decreases the bone density (long term effects of osteoporosis), retrieval of stored long term memory.

Increase in cortisol release causes the division of energy away from the low priority activities (such as the immune system) in order to survive the immediate thread/stress. Adrenal Fatigue impaired cognitive performance, dampened thyroid function, sleep disruption, decreased muscle mass, elevated blood pressure, lowered immune function, slow wound healing, increased abdominal fat, which has a stronger correlation to certain health problems than fat deposited in other areas of the body. Some of the health problems associated with increased stomach fat are heart attacks, strokes, higher levels of "bad" cholesterol (LDL) and lower levels of "good" cholesterol (HDL), which can lead to other health problems. http://www.adrenalfatigue.org/cortisol-adrenal-function. It disrupts the immune system, the enzyme balance, increase the blood pressure, increase the CRH due to the feed back of the corticotrophin secretion. Cortisol counteracts the insulin production, the blood sugar imbalances, and increases the hyperglycemia, gastric secretion, renal secretion, and acts as an antidiuretic, where the kidney produces 'hypotonic urine', and disrupts the breaking down of fats. Cushings syndrome is caused due to chronic stress, where cortisol secretion is excessive and prolonged. Addison's disease may be due to low levels of cortisol.

(Sources: Page 284-7)

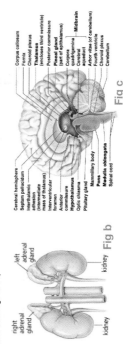

right adrenal gland

left adrenal gland

kidney   Fig b   kidney

Cerebral hemisphere
Septum pellucidum
Interthalamic
adhesion
(intermediate
mass of thalamus)
Interventricular
foramen
Anterior
commissure
Hypothalamus
Optic chiasma
Pituitary gland

Corpus callosum
Fornix
Choroid plexus
Thalamus
(encloses third ventricle)
Posterior commissure
Pineal gland
(roof of epithalamus)
Corpora
quadrigemina — Midbrain
Cerebral
aqueduct
Arbor vitae (of cerebellum)
Cerebellum
Mammillary body   Fourth ventricle
Pons   Choroid plexus
Medulla oblongata
Spinal cord

Fig c

APPENDIX G

Holmes and Rahe Stress Scale

Holmes and Rahe found that a score of 150 over 12 months gives you a 50–50 chance of developing an illness. A score of 300+ gives you a 90% chance of developing an illness, having an accident or "blowing up". Notice that "positive times" like Christmas, marriage and vacations are stressful.

LIFE EVENT (STRESSOR)	VALUE	#/YR		TOTAL
Death of spouse	100	X	=	
Divorce	73	X	=	
Marital separation	65	X	=	
Jail term	63	X	=	
Death of a close family member	63	X	=	
Major personal injury or illness	53	X	=	
Marriage	50	X	=	
Fired from work	47	X	=	
Marital reconciliation	45	X	=	
Retirement	45	X	=	
Major change in health of family member	44	X	=	
Pregnancy	40	X	=	
Sex difficulties	39	X	=	
Gain of new family member	39	X	=	
Major business readjustment	39	X	=	
Major change in financial state	38	X	=	
Death of close friend	37	X	=	
Change to different line of work	36	X	=	

LIFE EVENT (STRESSOR)	VALUE	#/YR		TOTAL
Major change in number of arguments with spouse	35	X	=	
Mortgage over $100,000	31	X	=	
Foreclosure of mortgage or loan	30	X	=	
Major change in responsibilities at work	29	X	=	
Son or daughter leaving home	29	X	=	
Trouble with in-laws	29	X	=	
Outstanding personal achievement	28	X	=	
Spouse begins or stops work	26	X	=	
Begin or end school	26	X	=	
Major change in living conditions	25	X	=	
Revision of personal habits	24	X	=	
Trouble with boss	23	X	=	
Major change in work hours or conditions	20	X	=	
Change in residence or schools	20	X	=	
Major change in recreation	19	X	=	
Major change in church activities	19	X	=	
Major change in social activities	18	X	=	
Mortgage or loan less than $10,000	17	X	=	
Major change in sleeping habits	16	X	=	
Major change in number of family get-togethers	15	X	=	
Major change in eating habits	15	X	=	
Vacations, Christmas	13	X	=	
Minor violations of the law	11	X	=	
			YOUR TOTAL	

(Source: Homes, T.H. and R.H. Rahe. "The Social Adjustment Rating Scale"; *Journal of Psychosomatic Research* (1967), 2:213–18.)

APPENDIX H

The Effects of Stress

Physical or mental stresses may cause physical illness
as well as mental and emotional problems.
Here are the parts of the body most affects by stress.

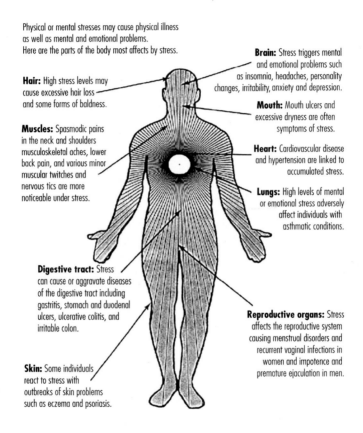

Brain: Stress triggers mental
and emotional problems such
as insomnia, headaches, personality
changes, irritability, anxiety and depression.

Hair: High stress levels may
cause excessive hair loss
and some forms of baldness.

Mouth: Mouth ulcers and
excessive dryness are often
symptoms of stress.

Muscles: Spasmodic pains
in the neck and shoulders
musculoskeletal aches, lower
back pain, and various minor
muscular twitches and
nervous tics are more
noticeable under stress.

Heart: Cardiovascular disease
and hypertension are linked to
accumulated stress.

Lungs: High levels of mental
or emotional stress adversely
affect individuals with
asthmatic conditions.

Digestive tract: Stress
can cause or aggravate diseases
of the digestive tract including
gastritis, stomach and duodenal
ulcers, ulcerative colitis, and
irritable colon.

Reproductive organs: Stress
affects the reproductive system
causing menstrual disorders and
recurrent vaginal infections in
women and impotence and
premature ejaculation in men.

Skin: Some individuals
react to stress with
outbreaks of skin problems
such as eczema and psoriasis.

(Source: The American Institute of Stress (AIS)
http://www.stress.org.)

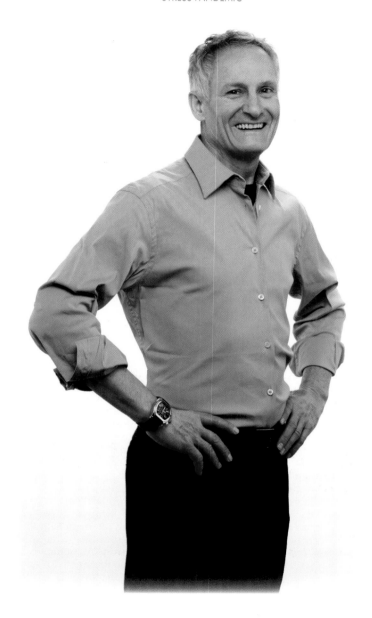

About the Author

Paul Huljich co-founded Best Corporation, a pioneering organic foods company listed on the stock exchange, of which he was chairman and joint-CEO. In leading the company to great success, during which its value grew to more than $100 million, Huljich gradually developed a number of stress-related conditions, including anxiety and depression. In 1998, as a result of years of culminated unchecked stress since he was a teenager, he experienced an overdose of chronic stress, which precipitated into a complete mental breakdown, losing his rights as a citizen and was made a ward of the state. He lost a lifetime of hard work. The consequences of which was disastrous to him and his immediate family.

Despite seeking the best care available, Huljich was informed by eleven psychiatrists that there was no cure for his illness, and that he would inevitably relapse, he felt like a broken man. Determined to free himself of his conditions, he began a comprehensive search globally for answers, as to why this happened to him. He traveled to the world-renowned Mayo Clinic in Minnesota and voluntarily admitted himself to the Menninger Clinic in Kansas for treatment.

Aided by exhaustive research, Huljich ultimately succeeded in fortifying himself and conquering his stress. He was able to overcome his debilitating condition, master stress and accomplish a healthy, positive way of life, naturally. He developed the nine-step 30 day Life Restyle Process to break the cycle of stress and achieve a unique LifeRestyle Solution, an overall wellness plan to live stress-free and thrive.

Since the year 2000, Huljich has not taken any medication related to any condition of the mind, nor has he suffered any relapse or needed any further treatment regarding any kind of mental illness. He has fully cured himself and has never felt better. He has great joy in his life and found his lost contentment.

Today he is back, better and stronger than before. He feels like a battle scarred warrior. He shares his hard won personal secrets and story, his struggle, his difficulties and finally his path to complete recovery and optimum wellness in *Stress Pandemic (Ed2): 9 Natural Steps to Break the Cycle of Stress and Thrive*.

Huljich is now one of America's top stress experts, a renowned public speaker, a stress management and LifeReStyle coach and a member of the American Institute of Stress.

He is also the author of the psychological thriller *Betrayal of Love and Freedom*. He has appeared in over 600 national and international radio shows, makes regular television and press appearances, while also blogging for *Psychology Today* and conducting motivational stress-free seminars.

Huljich is the father of three sons: Mark, Simon and Richard. He resides in New York City for most of the year and visits his homeland, New Zealand, regularly.

www.StressPandemic.com
www.LifeReStyle.org